Toward a
Restraint-Free Environment

This book is printed on recycled paper.♲

Toward a Restraint-Free Environment
Reducing the Use of Physical and Chemical Restraints in Long-Term and Acute Care Settings

edited by

Judith V. Braun, R.N., Ph.D.
Associate Administrator
Hebrew Home of Greater Washington
Rockville, Maryland

and

Steven Lipson, M.D., M.P.H.
Medical Director
Hebrew Home of Greater Washington
Rockville, Maryland
and
Associate Professor
Georgetown University School of Medicine
Washington, DC

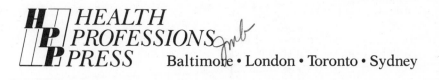

HEALTH PROFESSIONS PRESS Baltimore • London • Toronto • Sydney

Health Professions Press
P.O. Box 10624
Baltimore, Maryland 21285-0624

Typeset by Brushwood Graphics, Inc., Baltimore, Maryland.
Manufactured in the United States of America by
The Maple Press Company, York, Pennsylvania.

Library of Congress Cataloging-in-Publication Data
Toward a restraint-free environment : reducing the use of
  physical and chemical restraints in long-term and acute
  care settings / edited by Judith V. Braun, Steven Lipson.
      p.   cm.
  Includes bibliographical references and index.
  ISBN 1-878812-12-2
  1. Nursing home patients—Restraint.   2. Restraint of
patients.   3. Behavior therapy for the aged.   I. Braun, Judith V.,
1952–   . II. Lipson, Steven.
  [DNLM: 1. Long-Term Care.   2. Psychotropic Drugs.
3. Restraint, Physical.   WX 162 T737 1993]
RC954.3.T68   1993
610.73′61–dc20
DNLM/DLC   NWST   92-48379
for Library of Congress   1 AG M5970   CIP

(British Library Cataloguing-in-Publication data are
available from the British Library.)

Contents

Contributors

Judith V. Braun, R.N., Ph.D.
Associate Administrator
Hebrew Home of Greater
   Washington
6121 Montrose Road
Rockville, MD 20852

Patricia Carter, P.T., B.S.
Assistant Administrator
Hebrew Home of Greater
   Washington
6121 Montrose Road
Rockville, MD 20852

Renee Clermont, R.N., M.S., C.S.
Geropsychiatric Clinical Nurse
   Specialist
Hebrew Home of Greater
   Washington
6121 Montrose Road
Rockville, MD 20852

Jiska Cohen-Mansfield, Ph.D.
Director
Research Institute
Hebrew Home of Greater
   Washington
6121 Montrose Road
Rockville, MD 20852

**Barbara D. Fleischmann, B.S.,
C.T.R.S., L.N.H.A.**
Associate Administrator of
   Program Services
Margaret Wagner House of The
   Benjamin Rose Institute
2373 Euclid Heights Blvd.
Cleveland, OH 44106

J. Dermot Frengley, M.D., Ch.B.
Medical Director
Cohen Memorial Hospital
Roosevelt Island, New York 10044

**Mary Macholl Kaufmann, R.N.,
M.S.N.**
Instructor of Gerontological
   Nursing
Frances Payne Bolton School of
   Nursing
Case Western Reserve University
Cleveland, OH 44106
Director of Nursing
Margaret Wagner House of The
   Benjamin Rose Institute
2373 Euclid Heights Blvd.
Cleveland, OH 44106

Vivian J. Koroknay, R.N.C., M.S.
Gerontological Clinical Nurse
   Specialist
Hebrew Home of Greater
   Washington
6121 Montrose Road
Rockville, MD 20852

Steven Lipson, M.D., M.P.H.
Medical Director
Hebrew Home of Greater
   Washington
6121 Montrose Road
Rockville, MD 20852
Associate Professor
Georgetown University School of
   Medicine
Washington, DC 20057

Lorraine C. Mion, Ph.D., R.N.
Assistant Professor and
   Gerontological Nursing
   Specialty Coordinator
Medical-Surgical Program
Yale University School of Nursing
25 Park Street
New Haven, CT 06515

Proskauer Rose Goetz &
Mendelsohn
1233 Twentieth Street, N.W.
Suite 800
Washington, DC 20036-2396

Jeanne R. Samter, R.N., M.S.N.,
C.S.
Mental Health Coordinator
Hebrew Home of Greater
Washington
6121 Montrose Road
Rockville, MD 20852

Barbara E. Van Hala, M.Ed.,
C.T.R.S., O.C.L.P.
Director of Resident Programs
Columbus Park Chalet
6055 Bear Creek Drive
Bedford Heights, OH 44146

Perla Werner, M.A.
Research Associate
Research Institute
Hebrew Home of Greater
Washington
6121 Montrose Road
Rockville, MD 20852

May L. Wykle, Ph.D., R.N., FAAN
Director
CWRU Center on Aging and Health
Florence Cellar Professor and Chair
of Gerontological Nursing
Frances Payne Bolton School of
Nursing
Case Western Reserve University
Cleveland, OH 44106

Preface

In 1987, one of our nurse managers returned from a conference full of enthusiasm for a "new" approach to caring for nursing facility residents that involved minimal or no use of physical or chemical restraints. We knew of the passage of the Nursing Home Reform Act (OBRA '87), and some of us had visited facilities in England where restraints were not used and had attended conferences about the dangers of restraints. Despite this knowledge and our commitment to restorative care, we found the thought of changing the policies and practices of a 550-bed facility that had existed for more than 75 years and that employed many experienced staff overwhelming. In our experience, it had been much easier to implement a different care philosophy in a new facility than to change long-established habits. However, since this nurse manager was experienced in managing behavior problems, we thought she might be successful, and encouraged her to go ahead and see what happened. Within a year, we had our first 35-bed restraint-free unit.

Two years later, with the implementation of OBRA '87 looming before us, we had learned that change was possible and began institution-wide planning and implementation following the steps described in this book. At the start, we had 177 residents in physical restraints. We now have only 20. During this same period, we have significantly reduced the number of residents on antipsychotic and anxiolytic drugs. Although the transition has required a great deal of effort on the part of many staff, we believe it has resulted in better care and better staff morale. The "front-line" staff have been challenged to solve problems, not just to follow established procedures.

We had the advantage of time to learn and experiment, and access to resources not available to many care facilities across the country. We believe that the lessons we gleaned may make it easier for others to reduce the use of restraints in their facilities. Our book offers some pragmatic approaches to planning, organizing, and implementing a restraint reduction program. Although this book is based on our experiences in long-term care, we believe that much of the information it contains is equally applicable in the acute care facility. Likewise, the ideas and concepts presented in Chapter 8, "Physical Restraints in the Hospital Setting," are also germane to long-term care facilities.

Restraint reduction is the responsibility not only of the nursing and medical staffs, but of the full interdisciplinary team. All must be involved in the process of change. We hope that this book will be helpful to clinicians, including nurses, physicians, social workers, and physical and occupational therapists who care for older adults in a variety of settings, as well as to administrators who are seeking to implement or enhance restraint reduction and restorative care programs.

In truth, we write for ourselves and for other caregivers who have felt distressed by having to apply restraints or drug residents to lethargy for lack of alternatives. We expect that the patient rights and long-term care facility reform movements will continue to challenge us to find better ways to care for frail and disabled people, and that some of our readers will have lessons to teach us in the future.

Acknowledgments

A special thanks to all those at the Hebrew Home who persevered through the trial and error of implementing a restraint reduction program. We especially recognize the nurses and nursing assistants and the therapy staff who were open to creative approaches and continually demonstrated heartfelt caring.

This book could not have been completed without the assistance of Joyce Medlock. Her conscientious hard work, skillful word processing, and sensitive humor were invaluable.

Toward a
Restraint-Free Environment

Part I

Planning for and Creating a Restraint-Free Environment

Chapter 1

An Overview of Restraint Use and the Movement To Reduce the Use of Restraints

May L. Wykle

For decades, older adults in the United States were routinely restrained by both physical and chemical restraints. Although some of the use of restraints was legitimate, much abuse took place. Today, the use of chemical and physical restraints in the care of older adults is a matter of grave concern in long-term care facilities. How to manage older adults whose behavior requires continuous monitoring while at the same time preserving their dignity and autonomy represents one of the most difficult challenges for long-term care nursing; maintaining the independence and self-esteem of the frail older resident is a problem for the entire nursing home staff. Thanks to legislative initiatives and the activism of reformers, many long-term care facilities and other health care institutions are looking for alternatives to restraints that will enable these dual objectives to be met.

THE MOVEMENT TO REDUCE THE USE OF PHYSICAL AND CHEMICAL RESTRAINTS

In the 1980s, a reform movement to "untie the elderly" in nursing homes began. That movement spurred—and was in turn spurred by—the passage of the Omnibus Budget Reconciliation Act (OBRA) of 1987, which provides federal guidelines on the use of restraints with older adults in nursing homes. The interpretative guidelines to the OBRA regulations state that a nursing home resident has a right to be free of restraints and that physical restraints may be imposed

3

only if required for the treatment of the resident, and not for the purpose of discipline or the convenience of staff. As the movement to reduce the use of restraints in long-term care facilities gained momentum in the 1980s and 1990s, its message was carried beyond nursing homes to health care professionals in acute care and psychiatric hospitals.

The use of restraints in long-term care facilities has come under scrutiny partly because of a growing commitment to improving the quality of care and quality of life for nursing home residents (Blakeslee, 1988; Stilwell, 1988). Blakeslee (1988) has been zealous in her appeal to nursing homes to free older residents from restraints. She has demonstrated that restraints can be removed without jeopardizing nursing home residents' safety or adding staff. Her studies and those of other researchers (Kendal Corporation, 1990; McHutchion & Morse, 1989) have revealed the positive effects of removing restraints.

The movement to reduce the use of restraints in long-term and acute care settings has been at least partly effective. More and more professionals are speaking out against the use of restraints, and more and more nursing homes are reducing the number of residents they restrain. Nevertheless, every day in the United States more than 500,000 older adults are tied to their beds or chairs, in hospitals and nursing homes (Health Care Financing Administration, 1988; Lewin, 1989). Much work thus remains to be done in reducing the use of restraints in all care settings.

PREVALENCE OF RESTRAINTS

Physical restraint of older adults is common in nonpsychiatric settings in the United States (Frengley & Mion, 1986; Katz, Weber, & Dodge, 1981; Robbins et al., 1987). In acute care settings, prevalence is as high as 17%. In nursing homes, the prevalence is estimated at 19%–85% (Dube & Mitchell, 1986).

The prevalence of chemical restraints is high in long-term care settings, even though the use of psychotropic drugs is often inappropriate (Jencks & Clauser, 1991). Psychotropic drugs are often prescribed for reasons other than treating psychiatric diagnoses, including the chemical restraint of residents.

REASONS FOR USING RESTRAINTS

The only legitimate reason for using restraints is therapeutic—that is, to ensure the safety and well-being of the resident or patient. There is strong evidence to suggest, however, that restraints are often used for other reasons, including punishment of residents and the convenience of staff. Recent studies (Evans & Strumpf, 1989; Frengley & Mion, 1986) confirm that physical and chemical restraints are overused in both hospitals and nursing homes. Restraints are more likely to be overused when staff are not familiar with alternative forms of care. (Activities and behavior management as alternatives to the use of restraints are examined in Chapters 12 and 14.)

Despite the deleterious physical, mental, and emotional effects of restraints on residents (and sometimes on staff, who feel guilty about restraining frail older people), nursing home administrators often justify their use on the grounds that long-term care facilities are liable to be sued for damages should an unrestrained resident be hurt. This fear seems groundless. According to Francis (1989), nursing homes are more likely to be sued by families of residents who suffer as a result of being restrained than they are by families of residents who injure themselves while unrestrained. (For a full discussion of the legal issues surrounding the use of restraints, see Chapter 15.)

Use of Physical Restraints

Physical restraints are mechanical devices that limit a person's ability to function. They include wheelchair restraints, belts, side rails, and gerichairs. Historically, physical restraints have been used for a variety of reasons. In the late eighteenth century, Benjamin Rush (1745–1813), the father of the humanitarian movement in psychiatry in the United States, invented the tranquilizing chair. Mental patients were strapped into this chair for long periods of time, during which it was believed their mental stability would be restored. Rush also designed a gyrating device in which patients were bound upside down on a slanted, rotating wooden board. Both of these devices were believed to cure certain mental illnesses.

The lack of therapeutic value of restraints has been recognized for many decades. Nevertheless, residents of long-term care facilities continue to be restrained with devices not unlike Rush's tranquilizer chair. In many cases, the inability to manage psychiatric behavior has led to the use of restraints, even though researchers have documented that physical restraints often increase rather than calm agitated behavior (Gerdes, 1968; Werner, Cohen-Mansfield, Braun, & Marx, 1989). Other purposes for which restraints have been used by well-meaning caregivers include the prevention of assaultive behavior, wandering, falls, and poor posture, and the administration of medical treatment.

Several studies have polled nurses to try to determine why they believe they use restraints (Mion, Frengley, Jakovcic, & Marion, 1989; Strome, 1988; Strumpf & Evans, 1988; Yarmesch & Sheafor, 1984). These studies reveal that a majority of nurses are not opposed to using physical and/or chemical restraints if the resident's or patient's behavior warrants their use. Yarmesch and Sheafor (1984) presented nurses with several vignettes about restraining older adults. They elicited 149 different reasons for using restraints, among which protecting the patient and protecting other patients were the two most common reasons given. The wide variation in responses, however, suggests that restraints are not always used therapeutically, and that nurses have difficulty determining what behavior warrants the use of physical restraints.

Strumpf and Evans (1988) reported that the primary reasons for using restraints were the patient's confused mental status and the fear that the patient would fall if not restrained. In addition to polling caregivers, Strumpf and Evans asked patients why they thought they had been restrained. Interestingly, none of the patients stated that restraints were used to ensure effective treatment or to maintain medical therapies.

Mion et al. (1989) studied nurses on acute medical units and found that more than one reason was given for restraining 46% of the patients who were restrained. Some of the reasons given were: to maintain therapies, to prevent disruption of tubes and dressings, to manage wandering and wild behavior, and to maintain the patient's sitting balance. Strome (1988) found that physical restraints were used to control behavior that was violent or assaultive, or to restrain patients who were sensitive to psychotropic drugs and were not candidates for other types of therapy, such as behavior management.

Regrettably, restraints have been used for reasons other than those cited by these studies. Staff often find it easier to restrain residents than to supervise them. Restraints have also been used to punish residents. Even when restraints are not intended as a form of punishment, they are often viewed as such by residents. This stands to reason, since mechanical devices such as shackles, chains, and leather straps have long been used as forms of punishment. A resident who is restrained suffers from a loss of self-esteem and trust, and has difficulty accepting that he or she is benefiting by being restrained. To sever the connection between restraint use and punishment, caregivers should avoid linking the removal of the restraint with an improvement in behavior, a connection that reinforces the link between restraints and punishment. Instead, caregivers should encourage residents to regain control of their behavior, emphasizing their ability to be responsible.

Use of Chemical Restraints

As a result of the deinstitutionalization movement of the 1960s, many former mental patients were admitted to nursing homes. For the most part, staff did not know how to handle these residents' behaviors. Little training in caring for this new group of residents was provided, and staff were left with a difficult group of residents they did not understand. As a result, staff often relied on the medications that these new residents had used before they entered the nursing homes. This indiscriminate use of psychotropic drugs is now viewed as having been abusive. Unfortunately, these abuses have since tended to cloud the fact that psychotropic drugs have an important role to play in the care of some older nursing home residents, as shown in Chapter 10.

Parameters for the use of psychotropic drugs must be clearly identified and agreed upon by the treatment team, and the psychological effects, including side effects, of all psychotropic medications used in the nursing home need to be understood. A complete discussion of these issues appears in Chapter 10.

A MODEL FOR USING
PHYSICAL AND CHEMICAL RESTRAINTS

Physical and chemical restrains should be used only after alternatives are ruled out and resident outcomes considered. Wykle proposed a model for physical and chemical restraint use in older adults that considers the characteristics of the nurse, patient, and environment, on the one hand, and patient outcomes, on the other (Figure 1.1). The model presents a range of nurse characteristics that enter into the decision to use restraints or seek other alternatives. Characteristics of patients include their mental and physical status, age, behavior, and sensitivity to medication. The model also addresses such issues as availability of staff, medication used, administrative guidelines, and family preferences. The model can be used by nurses as a flow chart for making decisions about using restraints and for analyzing why restraints were used.

CONCLUSION

In the eighteenth century, Pinel sought humane treatment of people with mental illness. In the same tradition, advocates for older adults now seek better treatment of nursing home residents, many of whom are treated abusively. Health care professionals continue to be chal-

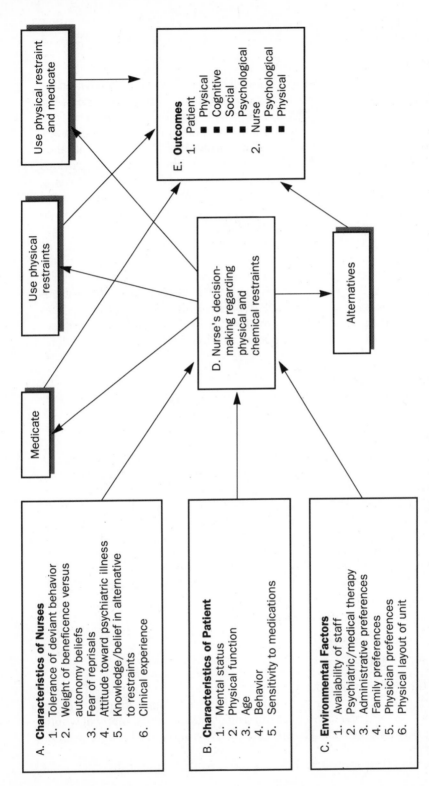

A. Characteristics of Nurses
1. Tolerance of deviant behavior
2. Weight of beneficence versus autonomy beliefs
3. Fear of reprisals
4. Attitude toward psychiatric illness
5. Knowledge/belief in alternative to restraints
6. Clinical experience

B. Characteristics of Patient
1. Mental status
2. Physical function
3. Age
4. Behavior
5. Sensitivity to medications

C. Environmental Factors
1. Availability of staff
2. Psychiatric/medical therapy
3. Administrative preferences
4. Family preferences
5. Physician preferences
6. Physical layout of unit

D. Nurse's decision-making regarding physical and chemical restraints

Alternatives

Use physical restraint and medicate

Use physical restraints

Medicate

E. Outcomes
1. Patient
   - Physical
   - Cognitive
   - Social
   - Psychological
2. Nurse
   - Psychological
   - Physical

Figure 1.1. Conceptual model of the decision-making process governing use of physical and chemical restraints. (Adapted from Wykle, 1989.)

8

lenged to find the least restrictive and most therapeutic interventions that enable them to provide safe care for nursing home residents while preserving their dignity and autonomy. More research must be done to investigate alternatives to physical and chemical restraints with older adults and to identify the benefits of reducing the use of restraints. Ethical issues, investigated in Chapter 16, also need to be examined more closely.

REFERENCES

Blakeslee, J.A. (1988). Untie the elderly. *American Journal of Nursing, 88,* 833–834.

Bornstein, P.E. (1985). The use of restraints on a general psychiatric unit. *Journal of Clinical Psychiatry, 46,* 175–178.

Dube, A.H., & Mitchell, E.K. (1986). Accidental strangulation from vest restraints. *Journal of the American Medical Association, 256,* 2275–2726.

Evans, L.K. (1989). *Restraint use with the elderly patient.* First National Conference on Nursing Research and Clinical Management of Alzheimer's Disease, University of Minnesota.

Evans, L.K., & Strumpf, N.E. (1989). Tying down the elderly. A review of the literature on physical restraint. *Journal of the American Geriatric Society, 37,* 65–74.

Federal Register. (1989). Rules and regulations, 54, 5317–5318.

Francis, J. (1989). Using restraints in the elderly because of fear of litigation. *New England Journal of Medicine, 320,* 870–871.

Frengle, J.D., & Mion, L.C. (1986). Incidence of physical restraints on acute general medical wards. *Journal of the American Geriatric Society, 34,* 565–568.

Gerdes, L. (1968). The confused or delirious patient. *American Journal of Nursing, 68,* 1228–1232.

Health Care Financing Administration. (1988). *Medicare/Medicaid nursing home information, 1987–1988.* Washington, DC: Department of Health and Human Services.

Jencks, S. (1985). Recognition of mental distress and diagnosis of mental disorder in primary care. *Journal of the American Medical Association, 253,* 1903–1907.

Jencks, S.F., & Clauser, S.B. (1991). Managing behavior problems in nursing homes. *Journal of the American Medical Association, 265*(4), 502–503.

Katz, L. Weber, F., & Dodge, P. (1981). Patient restraint and safety vests. *Dimensions of Health Service, 58,* 10–11.

Kendal Corporation. (1990). *Untie the elderly.* Kennet Square, PA: Author.

Lewin, T. (1989, December 28). Nursing homes rethink merits of tying the aged. *New York Times,* p. A1.

McHutchion, E., & Morse, J. (1989). Releasing restraints—a nursing dilemma. *Journal of Gerontological Nursing, 15*(2), 16–21.

Mion, L.C., Frengley, J.D., Jakovcic, C.A., & Marion, J.A. (1989). A further exploration of the use of physical restraints in hospitalized patients. *Journal of the American Geriatrics Society, 37,* 949–956.

Ray, W.A., Federspeil, C.F., & Schaffner, W. (1980). A study of antipsychotic drug use in nursing homes: Epidemiologic evidence suggesting misuse. *American Journal of Public Health, 37,* 485–491.

Robbins, L.J., Boyko, E., Lane, J., Cooper, D., & Jahnigen, D.W. (1987). Binding the elderly: A prospective study of the use of mechanical restraints in an acute care hospital. *Journal of the American Geriatrics Society, 34*(4), 290–296.

Soloff, P.H. (1978). Behavioral precipitants of restraint in the modern milieu. *Comparative Psychiatry, 19,* 179–184.

Stilwell, E.M. (1988). Use of physical restraints on older adults. *Journal of Gerontological Nursing, 14,* 42–43.

Strome, T.M. (1988). Restraining the elderly. *Journal of Psychosocial Nursing, 26*(9), 18–21.

Strumpf, N.E., & Evans, L.L. (1988). Physical restraint of the hospitalized elderly. Perceptions of the patients and nurses. *Nursing Research, 37,* 132–137.

Use of restraints—federal standards. (1984). Washington, DC: Department of Health and Human Services.

Werner, P., Cohen-Mansfield, J., Braun, J., & Marx, M.S. (1989). Physical restraints and agitation in nursing home residents. *Journal of the American Geriatrics Society, 37*(12), 1122–1126.

Wykle, M.L. (1989). *Use of physical and chemical restraints with the elderly.* Paper presented at the meeting of the National Gerontological Conference, Anaheim, CA.

Yarmesch, M., & Sheafor, M. (1984). The decision to restrain. *Geriatric Nursing, 5,* 242–244.

Chapter 2

Preparing for Implementation

Judith V. Braun

The practice of physically restraining frail nursing home residents was considered an acceptable method of protection for years. Many disciplines, including nursing, endorsed this practice; administrators, physicians, therapists, and others recommended and supported the use of restraints. Given this cross-disciplinary endorsement, reducing the use of restraints in long-term care facilities must be a team effort. Moreover, restraint removal must take place within a larger restorative framework. Older patients and residents need much more than simply to have their restraints untied. They need to be helped to walk. They need to be encouraged. They need to be assisted to become as functional as possible. Hence, a restraint reduction program must represent only one part of a larger restorative approach to care.

Although the current literature recommends that care facilities reduce the use of restraints (Blakeslee, 1988; English, 1989; Mitchell-Pedersen, Edmond, Fingerote, & Powell, 1985), standards of practice are not easily changed. For the most part, caregivers have applied physical restraints out of a desire to protect patients and residents from injury. Therefore, education alone cannot be expected to change the practice. Ongoing administrative support, time for staff to experience successes with alternatives to restraints, and time to incorporate the new practice are also necessary to change restraint practices permanently.

MAKING THE TRANSITION

Reducing the use of restraints is a major shift that leaves most caregivers uneasy. Such anxiety and distress can be counter-productive

11

and can impede changes in restraint practices. When presented with the concept of reducing restraint use, many caregivers, particularly those on evening and night shifts, resist. They are concerned that resource staff to help them develop alternatives will not be available when a situation warranting restraints arises.

Resistance of this sort can be overcome gradually by reducing the use of restraints in a transition phase that precedes restraint-free care. At the beginning of this phase, a thorough assessment is conducted for each patient or resident whom the caregiver would traditionally have restrained. Alternatives are developed and implemented, so that physical and chemical restraints become a last resort instead of a first course of action.

The transition environment is consistent with the intent of the 1987 OBRA regulations, which state that

> the resident has the right to be free from any physical restraints imposed or psychoactive drug administered for purposes of discipline or convenience, and not required to treat the resident's medical symptoms. (Health Care Financing Administration [HCFA], 1989, p. 5363)

Reducing the use of restraints as a first step leaves in place a safety net for the caregiver who is concerned that he or she will not have adequate knowledge and support to develop alternatives, or that the alternatives will not work. This allays some of the anxiety caregivers feel about removing restraints, and thus reduces some of the resistance. Simply knowing that restraints are a possible last resort seems to rechannel resistive energy into creative thinking about alternatives. As the caregiver experiences success with alternatives, physical and chemical restraints become less and less attractive.

Planning for and implementing a restraint reduction program can be the impetus that encourages staff, residents, and administration to adopt or expand a restorative care philosophy. Restorative care means more than removing a person's restraints and encouraging him or her to develop full range of motion. As an overriding philosophy, it pervades every element of care and involves every department of a long term-care facility.

Reducing the use of restraints as part of a restorative care philosophy involves much more than custodial care. Residents must be encouraged to be as functional as possible and must be assisted to achieve their highest level of independence. An approach that focuses solely on removing restraints is narrow and limiting. A restorative care approach to reducing the use of restraints includes teaching staff to help all residents or patients maximize their abilities and improve or maintain their function. The key elements of such an approach include *individualized care,* an *interdisciplinary approach,* and *innovative thinking.*

Individualized care means assessing each resident or patient, restrained or unrestrained, and planning and implementing care that will enhance his or her function. One cannot safely remove the posey vest from someone who has been restrained for months and whose muscles have become weak from disuse without first implementing a phased-in program for gradual muscle strengthening and walking. However, a generic walking program is not the solution for all residents. Individualized goals and approaches are essential for a successful restraint reduction program and for implementation of a restorative care philosophy.

A coordinated interdisciplinary approach that orchestrates the delivery of many different services is essential to enhancing the physical, mental, emotional, and spiritual functioning of residents in long-term care settings. Since the use of restraints is traditionally viewed as a nursing intervention, it is easy to view restraint removal as a nursing problem. A restorative care philosophy, however, demands that every discipline and every department be involved. The needs of residents or patients are too complex and varied to be met by any single discipline. Restraint alternatives and restorative care surpass the scope of nursing care strategies developed for the individual and frequently involve changes in the facility's physical and social environment, family participation, and revision of organizational routines. Hence, housekeeping and maintenance workers are as essential to the health care team as the nurse, physician, social worker, and therapist.

Innovation is critical to the success of a restraint reduction program. Implementing such a program calls for moving from the known—applying a restraint—to the unknown—developing an alternative. Identifying individualized, function-enhancing alternatives to restraints requires a considerable amount of creativity and ingenuity. Individuals who work with older people quickly recognize that what works for one resident may not work for a similar resident, and that what works with one resident one day may not work with the same resident the next. Continual reevaluation and innovation are paramount.

Where does one start to implement a restraint reduction program? Planning can begin with designation of a coordinator. It is essential that this person be seriously committed to limiting restraints and that he or she not assume the task of coordinating the program merely because of an assignment to do so or because of an interest in complying with federal regulations. The coordinator should be a staff person in a position of authority, who has earned the respect of staff and who can function as a role model. In many facilities the coordinator is an administrator or director of nursing.

The coordinator's first task is to become familiar with the literature on the use of restraints. Reading articles and talking with staff in other facilities that have implemented restraint reduction programs will help acquaint the coordinator with the facts, attitudes, and issues related to removing restraints. Reading this book is also an excellent first step to reducing the use of restraints.

PLANNING

Phase I: Identifying the Current Status

Once a coordinator is assigned, the initial phase of planning involves determining how the facility currently uses restraints. Generally, it is helpful to identify what the facility is changing *from* before deciding what to change *to* in the new program. What types of physical restraints does the facility use? Approximately how many residents are restrained? How often are these residents restrained? What kinds of psychoactive drugs are used, and how often? This information gives some idea of how extensive the restraint reduction program may need to be. Planning also involves determining the staff's prevailing feelings and beliefs about restraints. Do most nurses resist the idea of limiting physical restraints? What about nursing assistants? What do the heads of the major clinical departments, the director of nursing, the medical director, and the social services director think about restraints? Can one expect resistance at every level, or are the majority of staff members open to the program? Who seems to be most positive about the concept of removing restraints?

This information can be gathered by means of informal discussions with staff at all levels, in all departments. A formal survey of staff is not necessary and could, in fact, be more disruptive than helpful. Staff often feel that they are voting for a particular change when they complete a survey and are discouraged when they do not receive what they requested. Informal discussions serve not only to test the waters and introduce the concept of restraint reduction but also to help identify staff who are most positive about such a program and who could help to initiate it.

As restraint reduction is discussed, staff who have used restraints freely in the past may feel guilty about having used restraints. It is important to stress that changing a practice, such as the use of restraints, does not necessarily mean that the old way was wrong. For many years, the use of physical restraints was an acceptable method of practice. However, clinical practice changes, to reflect advances in knowledge.

In the early development of the program it is helpful to distribute pertinent articles and regulatory information to clinical department directors, administrators, and others in the facility who will be closely involved. Articles may concern the use of chemical and physical restraints as well as the implementation of restraint reduction programs in other facilities. The list of suggested readings at the end of this book includes many articles that staff may find useful.

Preliminary discussions with administrators and members of the board of directors are also essential to the initial stage of planning. A restraint reduction program has clear implications for risk management. Because of these implications and the difficulties that can arise if families, physicians, or others oppose restraint reduction, the support of the board and the administration are critical to the program's success. Support is easiest to elicit if administrators and board members are involved in planning from the onset and are given clinical, legal, and economic information related to removal. The need to conform to OBRA regulations may be the sole impetus behind administrative and board support. Nonetheless, board members and administrators who are well informed about the clinical, regulatory, and legal implications of restraint removal will be prepared to respond positively to queries from family members, residents or patients, and staff.

Phase II: Selecting the Interdisciplinary Committee

Once informal discussions have been held, administrative and board support have been secured, and the coordinator has a sense of the current status of restraint use in the facility and the staff's feelings about removing restraints, an interdisciplinary committee can be developed. Removing restraints, both physical and chemical, cannot be accomplished easily or efficiently by one discipline. A restraint reduction program with a restorative care focus requires a team approach and should be perceived as a team responsibility.

The role of the interdisciplinary committee involves three tasks or responsibilities:

1. To develop policies and procedures governing physical restraints and psychoactive drugs

2. To develop an implementation plan for the restraint reduction program

3. To serve as a steering committee to set the tone for a restorative care approach and to review progress during implementation

The role of the committee as a clinical/administrative group is to draft policies, procedures, and an implementation plan that are subject to administrative approval. The approval process is detailed later in this chapter.

Since long-term care facilities differ in size and organizational structure, the size and composition of the interdisciplinary committee will vary from facility to facility. An interest in keeping the committee small enough to work efficiently may cause one facility to limit the number on the committee to 8–10 members. Another facility, interested in involving as many departments and staff as possible from the onset, may develop a large advisory committee. The climate, structure, and priorities of the organization must be reviewed in deciding on the size and composition of the initial interdisciplinary committee.

At a minimum, the committee should consist of the following individuals, or individuals with comparable responsibilities:

- Designated coordinator person
- Director of nursing
- Medical director
- Director of social services
- Directors of therapies (physical, occupational, and speech)
- Director of activities
- Psychiatric services representative (e.g., a geropsychiatric clinical nurse specialist, a consulting psychiatrist, or other professional who can offer expertise on psychoactive drugs and behavioral interventions)
- Administrator responsible for risk management
- Supervisory level nurse (e.g., an assistant director of nursing or a supervisor who has responsibility for the day-to-day operations of the nursing department)
- Unit level nurse (e.g., a nurse manager or a charge nurse who has management/supervisory responsibilities at the unit level)

Others who may be included or added depending on the individual facility are:

- Director of education or staff development
- Family member of a resident or patient
- Representative of resident council
- Director of volunteers
- Director of public relations
- Housekeeping manager
- Maintenance manager
- Nursing assistant

Although all departments in the care facility may be affected by a restraint reduction program, it is not feasible for a working committee to include all of them. A system of subcommittees may be used to augment either a large interdisciplinary advisory committee or a small working group. Departments such as maintenance and housekeeping, which are not directly involved in implementing the program, may be included on a large advisory committee or may be invited to meetings of a small working group on an ad hoc basis. If a subcommittee structure is used, these departments may be included on a subcommittee dealing with issues related to the facility's physical environment.

In addition to the recommendations of a large advisory committee and/or a smaller working committee, input from other staff members, such as nursing assistants, can be gathered during the committee work process. Committee members may be asked to share draft copies of policies and procedures with their staff to elicit staff input and involve them in the planning process. The more staff members are involved in the planning process, the greater the likelihood of successful implementation of the program.

Phase III: Developing Policies and Procedures

The interdisciplinary committee's first responsibility is to develop policies and procedures related to the use of physical restraints and psychoactive drugs. A starting point may be to review the existing policies on restraints and to discuss a philosophy about use. Does the facility wish to become totally free of restraints? Is the goal to provide the least restrictive environment possible? In the latter case, the use of some restraints may be acceptable and the intent of the policy is to reduce the use of restraints. Many facilities have chosen to reduce restraint use with the long-range goal of moving toward restraint-free care. Such a transition allows for a gradual introduction of change that is more readily accepted and longer lasting than an abrupt one.

Once the committee decides on the goal or general policy regarding restraints, the second task is to identify the procedures that are necessary to implement the policy. The procedures for physical restraints and psychoactive drugs, although similar in structure, are different in content. Hence, separate procedures must be developed. To implement a restraint reduction program, the committee must establish:

1. Procedure for removing physical restraints
2. Procedure for applying physical restraints
3. Procedure for monitoring therapeutic use of psychoactive drugs.

Procedure for Removing Physical Restraints The first step in developing a procedure for removing physical restraints is to define physical restraints. This definition can incorporate regulatory language and should be specific to the facility.

Physical restraints may be defined as:

> Any manual method or physical or mechanical device, material, or equipment attached or adjacent to the resident's body that the individual cannot remove easily which restricts freedom of movement or normal access to one's body. Physical restraints include, but are not limited to leg restraints, arm restraints, hand mitts, soft ties or vests, wheelchair safety bars, geri-chairs that prevent rising, and bedrails. (HCFA, 1992, p. 76)

Although the OBRA 1987 interpretive guidelines did not include siderails in its definition of physical restraints, subsequent drafts of the interpretive guidelines have included siderails. Misuse of bedrails involves using them to keep a resident from getting out of bed voluntarily. Hence, half-siderails that provide protection from rolling out of bed but that do not confine a resident are preferable to the more restrictive full or three-quarter rails. If siderails/bedrails are not included in the initial procedure statement, they may be addressed on an individual-by-individual basis during implementation. Unfortunately, most care facilities do not have funds readily available to replace all of their beds or even purchase half-siderails for all of their beds. However, if a facility is being built, or an old facility is being renovated, half-siderails should be considered. Residents who do not need siderails can be identified during the assessment process of implementation. For other residents who could benefit from lower beds or half-siderails, economically feasible alternatives may be implemented (see Chapter 6).

The procedure for removing physical restraints must include steps to identify residents in restraints, to assess each resident thoroughly, and to develop and implement alternative care plans. These steps ensure that the safety needs of each patient or resident are considered before his or her restraints are removed. Details for each of these steps are included in subsequent chapters. A multidisciplinary checklist, such as that shown in Figure 2.1, can be used to remind staff of the steps in the procedure and to document in the patient's or resident's record that each step was completed. The checklist might also include information on the type of restraint being removed and the frequency with which it was being used. Suggested steps to include in the checklist require staff to:

1. Identify the type of restraint/protective device used, when and how often it is used, and why it is used.

2. Request a consultation with the coordinator.

3. Request a consultation with the physical therapist as appropriate.

4. Request a consultation with the mental health professional as necessary.

5. Identify an alternative care plan.

6. Contact the family and the patient or resident to discuss an alternative care plan.

7. Contact the physician and have him or her rewrite an order to reflect the new care plan.

8. Document the alternative care plan on the existing care plan.

9. Discuss the care plan with staff on all three shifts.

The procedure for removing restraints should include a mechanism for communicating alternative care plans within the nursing department, particularly to nursing assistants on all three shifts. A sample procedure is shown in Table 2.1.

Procedure for Evaluating and Using Physical Restraints
Implementation of a restraint reduction program implies that physical restraints may still be used. The criteria for applying physical restraints and the process to follow while the restraints are in use should be delineated in a procedure statement. (A sample procedure for using physical restraints is shown in Table 2.2.)

The initial portion of the procedure statement for using restraints may be similar to the statement for removing them. The checklist may be used to document that the appropriate assessments were completed; alternative care plans were developed and tried; and that family, resident or patient, and physician were consulted. Applying physical restraints thus becomes the last resort when all else has failed.

□ Removing physical restraint
□ Considering physical restraint

Name: _____ Room# _____ Unit: _____

Reason for considering/using a physical restraint:

Falling □ Wandering □ Positioning □ Physical aggression □
Maintain medical treatment □ Change in functional ability □
Other □ (Specify _____)

Type of physical restraint currently used:

Chair belt □ Roll belt □ Vest □ Mittens □ Wrist ties □ Lap tray □
Toe loop □ Other □, specify _____

When is it used? Please specify how many hours per shift:
_____ day _____ evening _____ night
Please specify how many days a week: _____

Which of the following evaluations has been performed?

□ Nursing rehabilitation consultation   Date _____ Initials _____
□ Physical/occupational therapy evaluation   Date _____ Initials _____
   or wheelchair assessment
□ Mental health consultation   Date _____ Initials _____

Alternatives to restraint

□ Environmental:
Chair wedge □ Antitippers □ Antislip strips □ Other □, specify: _____
□ Physiological (Specify _____)
□ Psychosocial (Specify _____)
□ Activities (Specify _____)
□ Alterations in care (Specify _____)

Decisions

Remove restraint □ Continue to use restraint □ Apply restraint □
□ Reason for use: _____

Type of protective device to be used:
Chair belt □ Roll belt □ Vest □ Mittens □ Wrist ties □ Lap tray □
Toe loop □ Other □, specify _____

When is restraint to be used? Please specify how many hours per shift:

_____ day _____ evening _____ night
Please specify how many days a week: _____
□ Care plan changed   Date _____ Initials _____
□ Physician order changed   Date _____ Initials _____
□ Family/resident or patient notified   Date _____ Initials _____

Figure 2.1. Sample multidisciplinary checklist for physical restraints.

Table 2.1. Sample procedure statement for removing physical restraints

Policy

The _____ facility supports the belief that long-term care facility residents should live in the least restrictive setting possible. To preserve the dignity and autonomy of its residents and to provide quality life and health care, this facility does not use physical restraints or protective devices except when other alternatives are not appropriate.

Definitions

Physical restraints and protective devices: Any manual method or physical or mechanical device, material, or equipment attached or adjacent to the resident's body that the resident cannot remove easily and that restricts the person's freedom of movement or normal access to his or her own body. Physical restraints and protective devices include, but are not limited to, leg restraints, hand mitts, soft ties or vests, wheelchair safety bars, arm restraints, lap trays, toe loops, geri-chairs that prevent rising, and bedrails.

Procedure

Facility staff will:

I. Identify all residents with physical restraints.

II. Have the unit's team confer to complete a physical restraint checklist on each resident:

   a. Identify type of restraint/protective device used, when and how often it is used, and why it is used.

   b. Request and complete nursing rehabilitation consultation.

   c. Request and complete physical therapy consultation as necessary.

   d. Request and complete mental health consultation as necessary.

   e. Identify an alternative care plan.

   f. Contact family to discuss alternative care plan.

   g. Change physician order to reflect new care plan.

   h. Document alternative care plan on the existing care plan.

III. Retain original checklist on the chart.

IV. Discuss alternative care plan with staff on all three shifts.

V. Phase in the alternative care plans when the necessary equipment is available. Start with residents whose likelihood of success is greatest.

VI. Review nursing assistant assignments and make alterations as necessary to ensure adequate monitoring of residents.

Incorporating the checklist into the procedure statement for using restraints serves two purposes. First, it documents that alternatives were attempted and failed. Second, it forces the nurse to try alternatives first and seek help from other resources before automatically applying a restraint. Although physical restraints may be used in emergency circumstances, it is helpful to require that the steps

Table 2.2. Sample procedure statement for evaluating and using physical restraints

Policy

The _____ facility supports the belief that long-term care facility residents should live in the least restrictive setting possible. To preserve the dignity and autonomy of its residents and to provide quality life and health care, this facility does not use physical restraints or protective devices except when other alternatives are not appropriate.

Definitions

Physical restraints and protective devices: Any manual method or physical or mechanical device, material, or equipment attached or adjacent to the resident's body that the resident cannot remove easily and that restricts the person's freedom of movement or normal access to his or her own body. Physical restraints and protective devices include, but are not limited to, leg restraints, hand mitts, soft ties or vests, wheelchair safety bars, arm restraints, lap trays, toe loops, geri-chairs that prevent rising, and bedrails.

Procedure

Facility staff will:

I. Have the unit's team confer to complete a physical restraint checklist on each resident:

    a. Identify type of restraint/protective device used, when and how often it is used, and why it is used.

    b. Request and complete nursing rehabilitation consultation.

    c. Request and complete physical therapy consultation as necessary.

    d. Request and complete mental health consultation as necessary.

    e. Identify an alternative care plan.

    f. Contact family to discuss alternative care plan.

    g. Change physician order to reflect new care plan.

    h. Document alternative care plan on the existing care plan.

II. Institute the following, if the plan calls for using a protective device on a resident:

    a. Have the unit's team review the resident's need for a physical restraint at least every 7 days.

    b. Have the physician evaluate the resident at least every 7 days with nursing to determine the appropriateness of using a physical restraint. If indicated, have the order for a physical restraint rewritten. The order should specify the type of physical restraint to be used, as well as how often and for what purpose it is to be used.

    c. Reposition the resident at least every 2 hours, if necessary for the type of physical restraint used. A licensed person should enter documentation for the use of the physical restraint and repositioning in the treatment book during every shift.

    d. In an emergency situation when there is an immediate danger to the patient or resident or to others, apply a physical restraint, and have the appropriate order from a physician documented as soon as possible, but no later than within 1 hour. Initiate the physical restraint checklist within 1 working day.

described in the checklist be initiated within at least 24 hours of restraint application.

At a minimum, requirements to be met when a restraint is in use may consist of federal and state regulations governing the use of physical restraints. These may include:

1. A written physician's order noting the type of restraint, the circumstances under which the restraint may be used, and the specific period of time during which the restraint may be used
2. A specification for removal of the restraint every 2 hours to allow exercise, use of the toilet, and a check for skin redness.

Additional requirements may be added to ensure regular evaluation of the continued need for the restraint. Still other requirements may be included to ensure the judicious use of physical restraints and to provide disincentives for relying on such restraints. Suggestions for such requirements include:

1. A team review of the patient's or resident's need for a restraint at least every 7 days and documentation of the reasons for continued use of the restraint
2. A physician and nurse evaluation of the patient or resident at least every 7 days and, if the restraint continues to be indicated, a rewrite of the physician's order

A reevaluation period of more than 7 days can be used. However, a time frame of less than every 30 days is recommended, for three reasons. First, a resident's condition may change, and a lengthy time frame for reevaluation may result in the unnecessary use of a restraint for a prolonged period. This could easily result in immobility for the patient or resident. Second, physician orders commonly are renewed every month. When a reevaluation is required at the same time as the renewal of orders, the tendency is to renew orders for physical restraints automatically without conducting a thoughtful reevaluation of the patient or resident. Third, a requirement to reevaluate frequently and to rewrite the order for a physical restraint creates a burden on staff. Thus, the burden becomes an additional incentive to encourage staff members to identify creative alternatives.

Procedures for applying specific types of restraints used in the facility, such as geri-chairs, posey vests, wrist restraints, and the like, may be included in this procedure or addressed separately.

Procedure for Monitoring Use of Psychoactive Drugs Psychoactive drugs may be used therapeutically to treat specific psychiatric illnesses. At times, however, mind-altering drugs, such as tranquilizers, have been used in long-term care facilities and other settings as chemical restraints to control troublesome behaviors. As stated in the OBRA regulations, psychoactive drugs that are used for discipline or staff convenience are chemical restraints and hence are prohibited. However, an antipsychotic drug used to treat a patient or resident with manifestations of a diagnosed psychosis may be appropriate. Hence, all psychoactive drugs are not chemical restraints, and all such drugs should not be eliminated.

A procedure statement for monitoring the therapeutic use of psychoactive drugs is similar in structure to that for physical restraints. (A sample procedure statement is shown in Table 2.3.) However, the content of the statement and the individuals responsible for the steps it recommends will be different. The procedure statement should address the following areas:

1. How is a psychoactive drug defined?
    a. Will the procedure statement apply only to antipsychotics?
    b. Will the statement apply to stimulants, narcotics, antidepressants, anxiolytics, and sedative/hypnotics?
2. Assessment
    a. How will reviews be conducted?
    b. How often will reviews be conducted? Who will conduct them?
    c. How will behaviors be assessed and documented?
    d. How will side effects be assessed?
3. Interventions
    a. How will behavioral interventions be incorporated into the care plan?
    b. Who will determine the need for drug reductions, increases, and the like? The psychiatrist? The primary physician?

Approval of Policies and Procedures Many drafts of policy and procedure statements are often generated before the interdisciplinary committee can reach consensus on a final version. Although this process is time consuming and often produces conflict, soliciting staff input during the revision phases helps to involve staff in the planning and encourages their acceptance of the final procedure.

Depending on the facility's resources and policies, the committee's final version of the policy and procedure statement may be reviewed and approved by the following groups or individuals before implementation:

- Administrator
- President or representative of the board of directors

Table 2.3.   Sample procedure statement for monitoring use of psychoactive drugs

---

Policy
Psychoactive drugs are used only to treat a patient's or resident's specific medical symptoms. Patients or residents on psychoactive drugs are reviewed regularly. Suggestions for drug discontinuation, dose reductions, and/or behavior management alternatives are discussed at the review with the medical and nursing staff responsible for the patient's or resident's care.

Definitions
Psychoactive drugs: Drugs prescribed to control mood, mental status, or behavior. Types of drugs regularly reviewed include, but are not limited to:

- Stimulants
- Narcotics
- Antipsychotics
- Antidepressants
- Anxiolytics
- Sedatives and hypnotics

Procedure
Facility staff will:

I.   Conduct review of psychoactive drugs at least every 60–120 days on every patient or resident receiving psychoactive drugs as defined above.

II. Have the geropsychiatric clinical nurse specialist coordinate these rounds; include the consulting psychiatrist and, at a minimum, the primary medical and nursing providers on the unit.

III. Use pharmacy printouts to identify for review residents who are receiving the drugs listed above on each unit.

IV. At a minimum, address the following questions at the review:

   A.   Does the patient or resident have a condition that is appropriately treated with this drug?

   B.   If the drug is an antipsychotic, does the patient or resident have one of the following specific conditions documented in his or her medical record?

   1.   Schizophrenia
   2.   Schizoaffective disorder
   3.   Delusional disorder
   4.   Psychotic mood disorders (including mania and depression with psychotic features)
   5.   Acute psychotic episodes
   6.   Brief reactive psychosis
   7.   Schizophreniform disorder
   8.   Atypical psychosis
   9.   Tourette's disorder
   10. Huntington's disease

(continued)

Table 2.3. (continued)

---

11. Organic mental syndromes (including dementia and delirium) with associated psychotic and/or agitated behaviors:

   a. Which have been quantitatively (i.e., number of episodes) and objectively (e.g., biting, kicking, scratching) documented;

   b. Which are not caused by preventable reasons; and

   c. Which are causing the resident to:
   - Present a danger to herself or himself or to others,
   - *Continuously* cry, scream, yell, or pace if these specific behaviors cause *an impairment* in *functional capacity,* or
   - Experience psychotic symptoms (hallucinations, paranoia, delusions) not exhibited as dangerous behaviors or as crying, screaming, yelling, or pacing but which cause the resident distress or impairment in functional capacity.

12. Short-term (7-day) symptomatic treatment of hiccups, nausea, vomiting, or pruritus. (HCFA, 1992, pp. 147–148)

C. Is the drug effective as judged by a change in symptoms or behavior?

D. Is the patient or resident experiencing any side effects from the drug?

E. Should the drug dose be increased, decreased, or discontinued? Why?

V. Have the consulting psychiatrist document the review and any recommendations in the medical record.

Note: Part IV,B is based on the Interpretive Guidelines issued by the Health Care Financing Administration (1992).

- Legal counsel
- Insurance broker or carrier
- Resident care policy committee
- Quality assurance committee
- Risk management committee
- Mental health consultants
- Pharmacy consultants

Phase IV: Developing an Implementation Plan

The interdisciplinary committee's second task is to develop a plan for implementation. Such a plan should include specific tasks that must be accomplished, the time frame for completing those tasks, and the individuals responsible for them. Areas that should be addressed are education and marketing activities for staff, patients or residents and their families, outside physicians, and the community, as well as the actual implementation of these activities. Specifics regarding education and implementation are included in Chapters 3 and 4, respectively.

Once general education for facility-wide staff, patients or residents, and families is accomplished, actual implementation of a restraint reduction program is approached most successfully on a unit-by-unit basis. The order in which units will implement the program should be determined based on the number of restraints used on the unit and the readiness of staff. For optimal success, the first unit to implement the plan should be the one whose staff are most open to the concept of restraint reduction. The cooperation of the nurse manager and/or charge nurse is critical to the success of the program. One way to identify the unit that is most ready to initiate the program is to ask for volunteers to be the pioneer unit. A second method is to choose the unit that uses the fewest and perhaps easiest-to-remove restraints. Word within a facility travels quickly; success on the first unit will enhance the likelihood of success on subsequent units.

Once the start-up unit is identified, implementation activities on the unit follow this sequence:

1. The coordinator meets with all staff on the unit, including all departments (e.g., housekeeping, dietary, nursing, social services) on all three shifts to review information covered in general in-services, discuss the types of residents or patients on the unit, identify the components of the program and the procedures for implementation, and answer questions and concerns of the staff.

2. All residents or patients who are currently restrained are identified.

3. The first resident or patient who will have his or her restraints removed is selected, starting with those who are at the least risk for hurting themselves and who present the highest potential for success.

4. The remainder of the procedure is followed, including communication with the resident or patient, the family, and the physician; development and implementation of a restorative care plan; and ongoing evaluation and communication with staff.

Implementation on a single unit can take anywhere from 1 to 6 weeks to accomplish. Although the full restraint reduction program should be implemented on one unit at a time, parts of the program may be introduced on a limited basis to all units. Such an expansion of the program will depend on the coordinator's availability. The limited introduction may include requiring that the coordinator evaluate and assist the health care team in developing a restorative care plan for all newly admitted patients or residents and/or all of those whom the team determine to need a new order for restraints. Expanding the program to all units in this way introduces the restorative care concept gradually to staff and prevents the initiation of new restraint orders. Walking programs may also be initiated on units before the actual restraint reduction program is implemented. Walking helps to build muscle strength for restrained and unrestrained residents alike.

Phase V: Developing a Progress Review Mechanism

A steering committee is needed to review the progress of the program, resolve interdepartmental problems, and disseminate information on the outcomes and evaluation of the project. The interdisciplinary committee may serve as the steering committee or a new steering committee may be appointed. It is helpful to designate this committee before implementation begins. The frequency of the committee's meetings may be established by the committee itself or arranged on an as-needed basis during implementation.

Issues that may arise and could be addressed by the steering committee include the objections of families to the removal of restraints; environmental hazards, such as highly polished, slippery floors; and programming of activities to meet residents' or patients' restorative needs and unit routines. These issues involve many departments and require an interdisciplinary approach for resolution. Regular committee meetings will provide a structure for follow-up to ensure that communication occurs among departments, that responsibilities are assigned, and that problems are resolved.

In addition, the committee can identify outcome measures that will be used to evaluate the program's progress. The steering committee can monitor data on serious injuries, wandering incidents, and other pertinent outcomes to identify trends and problem areas. Additional suggestions for outcome measures are included in Chapter 9.

Finally, the steering committee can play a major role in continually reinforcing a restorative care approach. Although a restraint reduction program may reach completion when all restraints are removed, a restorative care approach is never-ending. With each new resident or patient who enters the facility and each new employee who joins the staff, a new restorative care challenge arises. In addition, residents or patients and staff members alike can benefit from continual encouragement and support to maintain a restorative care perspective. Facility policies, procedures, and practices require ongoing review and revision to remain current with new knowledge and trends for restorative care. An interdisciplinary steering committee can perform all of these functions and can be the mechanism for putting a restorative care philosophy into practice.

REFERENCES

Blakeslee, J.A. (1988). Untie the elderly, *American Journal of Nursing, 88*, 833–834.

English, R.A. (1989). Implementing a non-restraint philosophy. *The Canadian Nurse, 85*(3), 52–55.

Health Care Financing Administration. (1989). Conditions of participation and requirements for long term care facilities. *Federal Register, 54*(21), 5359–5373. Washington, DC: Government Printing Office.

Health Care Financing Administration. (April, 1992). Interpretive guidelines. *State Operations Manual*, Transmittal 250. Washington, DC: Government Printing Office.

Mitchell-Pedersen, L., Edmond, L., Fingerote, E., & Powell, C. (1985). Let's untie the elderly. *Quarterly Journal of Long Term Care, 21*(10), 10–14.

Chapter 3

Educating Staff, Residents, and Families About Restraint Reduction

Vivian J. Koroknay, Judith V. Braun, and Steven Lipson

Education is critical to the success of a restraint removal program. Everyone involved in the care of older adults, both directly and indirectly, needs to understand the philosophy and activities of a restorative care approach. Education provides knowledge, as well as a forum for problem-solving, communication, and team building. The educational needs of staff are different from those of patients or residents and families. This chapter examines educational programs and strategies for staff from all departments, patients or residents, family members, boards of directors, and physicians.

STAFF EDUCATION

Educating is the most important step in implementing a restraint reduction program. For years, restraint use has been the standard of care. A change from this standard makes staff members extremely anxious. A comprehensive educational program is essential to inform staff adequately and reduce their anxiety about the proposed change. Changing habits and practices is generally easier when people understand clearly what the changes will entail and what the end result will be. Disseminating information through educational programs and demonstrations will help the staff feel safer in making the change in policy and will encourage their support (Kanter, 1985).

A first step in the process of staff education is to designate a coordinator who will not only educate the staff but will continue to assist them as the program is implemented. The selection of such a person indicates administrative support of the program. The coordinator can play a pivotal role in steadying the disequilibrium that accompanies change by giving the nursing staff the hands-on assistance they will need to implement the program. A gerontological clinical nurse specialist is an excellent choice as coordinator of a restraint reduction program. With his or her advanced knowledge of aging and health, the clinical nurse specialist can facilitate the implementation of the program by educating all staff. The clinical nurse specialist can also provide the nursing staff with ongoing consultation and clinical demonstrations, which are vital to the success of the program.

If it is not possible to assign a clinical nurse specialist, an assistant director of nursing could be selected as the project coordinator. As has been noted in Chapter 2, the coordinator should be enthusiastic about reducing the use of restraints and should not be assigned for the sole purpose of complying with regulations. It is important to ensure that the coordinator will have adequate time to carry out the task, since the implementation process requires ongoing education and consultation.

Before the staff can recognize the benefits of reducing the use of restraints, their attitudes about using them must first change. This is an important part of the education process. According to Bennis and associates (cited in Chang, 1981), change involves three strategies. First is the power-coercive approach, which makes use of administrators' power to influence change. An example of this approach is the creation of a policy that restricts the use of restraints. Second is the rational-empirical approach to change. This strategy assumes that if those who are required to change are given adequate and appropriate information, change will take place. Education of staff regarding the dangers of restraint use and the benefits of restraint removal is part of this approach and often is done in the classroom. Third is the normative-reeducative approach, which assumes that change will take place when attitudes and values are changed. This change in values takes place at the individual and/or unit levels.

All members of the facility's staff are involved in the restraint reduction program, and all need education. Not only must all staff accept and feel comfortable with the possibility that residents may wander from their units, but all departments must cooperate if alternatives to restraints are to work. For instance, the placement of nonslip strips on the floors involves four departments: nursing staff first recognizes the need for strips in places where a resident slides frequently, such as in the bathroom; environmental services must clean the floor appropriately so the strips do not come off the floor;

engineering then places the strips; and administration must allow the staff time to implement this alternative.

General Inservice

A basic introduction to the concept of restraint reduction and the evolution of the new policy can be presented in a general inservice for all staff. The content outline for this session should include information on misconceptions about the use of restraints, the dangers of immobility, alternatives to restraints, and liability issues. The inservice is also a good time to address the guilt that some staff members may feel for having used restraints in the past. Offering reassurance that health care is always changing in response to new knowledge is one way to deal with this important issue.

The general inservice should be mandatory for all staff on all three shifts. Approximately 30 minutes should be allowed for the inservice. Because the amount of information to be covered is great, the teaching technique should be primarily lecture, with time allotted for questions and answers. However, additional teaching techniques should be used to solicit audience interest and participation. For instance, a video showing residents restrained in their chairs or beds in contrast to residents walking about freely offers an excellent opportunity to discuss the dangers of restraint use. A video that presents interviews with residents who have been restrained is also effective. Another technique is to put restraints on staff volunteers from the audience during the inservice and then have them describe how it felt to be tied up. A sample outline for the general inservice is shown in Table 3.1. Appendix 3.A is a sample of a handout that may be distributed to staff members during the meeting.

Unit Inservices

Staff members who provide direct care, nurses and nursing assistants in particular, need more education than can be provided at the mandatory inservice. This additional education is best accomplished in small groups, where staff members may feel more at ease in raising questions and expressing their concerns.

Small inservices can take place on individual units as each unit begins the restraint reduction process. These inservices should be conducted on all three shifts, and all staff, including the nursing staff, the activities staff, the dietitian, the dietary aide, and the social worker assigned to the unit, should be required to attend. These meetings should be used to inform the staff about the specific procedure their unit will follow in removing restraints. For instance, staff members will feel more comfortable if they know that re-

Table 3.1. Sample outline for general inservice on removing physical restraints

I. Introduction of new policy and procedure
    A. Hand out and review of new policy and procedure
        1. Procedure for removal of physical restraints
        2. Procedure for use of physical restraints
    B. Definition of physical restraint according to federal regulations and facility's policy

II. History of restraint use as an acceptable standard of care for
    A. Prevention of falls for frail older adults
    B. Prevention of wandering
    C. Dealing with agitated patients or residents who might present a danger to themselves or others

III. Reasons for removing restraints and changes in standards of care that accompany increased knowledge
    A. Devastating effects of immobility
        1. Changes in body systems
        2. Loss of functional ability, increased dependence on staff for activities of daily living
        3. Increased depression, withdrawal from surroundings, agitation
        4. Increased risk of serious injuries from falls
    B. Ethical issues and the resident's right to be free of restraints
    C. Risk of falls versus benefits of restraint removal

IV. Legal implications
    A. Accidental death and injury resulting from restraint use
    B. Facility's liability
    C. Federal mandate that residents have the right to be free of restraints
    D. Courts' inclination to accept an increased risk of falls in older adults

V. Overview of some general alternatives to restraints
    A. Restorative care
        1. Individualized care (care based on the resident's needs)
        2. Interdisciplinary care planning
        3. Maintenance of functional independence at whatever level is possible
    B. Meeting residents' physiological needs
        1. Ambulation/mobility/exercise/outdoor time
        2. Toileting
        3. Addressing increased needs during acute illness
    C. Environmental approaches
        1. Individualized seating
        2. Lowered beds, furniture rearranged for resident's safety
        3. Nonslip flooring
        4. Improved lighting
        5. Alarms
    D. Psychosocial approaches
        1. Activities
        2. Companionship
        3. Attention to individual needs

IV. Implementation
    A. Unit-by-unit basis/one restraint at a time
    B. Individual unit inservices
    C. Primary nursing assistant input
    D. Time allotment for observation of residents when restraints are removed

straints will be removed one at a time starting with the easiest cases first. This is also a good time to reassure staff members that they will be given adequate time to observe and assess residents' responses when the restraints are removed.

Unit inservices should provide detailed information on alternatives to restraints. This is an excellent opportunity to solicit nursing assistants' opinions about the residents with whom they are most familiar. For instance, the primary nursing assistants probably know which residents' restraints will be the easiest to remove. They will likely have insights about which alternatives might be most successful and what problems they can anticipate. Encouraging the nursing assistants to participate in establishing the restraint removal care plans reassures them that their ideas are a valuable part of the program. This, in turn, helps ensure the program's success.

During the unit inservices, it is important to establish a procedure for communicating the care plan for restraint removal. Restraint removal care plans tend to be complex, involving more than one alternative. A typical care plan may call for changes in seating requirements as well as establishment of a walking schedule and a toilet schedule. Furthermore, the requirements may differ for different shifts. The nursing assistant staff will need to know how they will learn about the care plan and what they are expected to do to follow it. Specific ways to communicate the plan to the staff members are found in Chapter 4. Both written and verbal communication are necessary to ensure that staff members understand the restraint reduction alternatives.

Ongoing Education

After the formal unit inservices, incidental teaching continues. Many residents will need close observation when a restraint is first removed. During this time, discussions with the nursing assistant staff not only provide insight into the effectiveness of the prescribed plan, but also allow the nursing assistant to raise any questions about the plan and note any problems with it. Answering questions and assisting with problem solving are essential parts of the educational process for those who provide direct care to residents and patients.

Once the restraint reduction program is in place, follow-up inservices will be needed. These inservices may cover topics related to restraint removal. One topic that usually needs review is proper wheelchair positioning for those patients or residents who need wheelchair adaptations to prevent them from sliding out of their chairs. Nursing staff may also need to discuss interventions for new patients or residents who were previously restrained, but are now admitted to a unit or nursing home with a restraint reduction program.

Ongoing instruction in assessment and prevention of falls is an almost constant need, since patients and residents experience physical changes and may deteriorate. Even those who were never restrained may need interventions to keep them from falling without resorting to restraints. Further education in restorative care is also needed. Topics for such programs might include walking and exercise programs, and programs for incontinence prevention programs. Appendix 3.B is a sample of a handout that may be distributed during a follow-up inservice.

Approximately a year after a restraint reduction program is initiated, the facility might repeat general inservices for the entire staff to help reinforce the program's philosophy. Two possible topics for general inservices are preventing falls and planning for restorative care. Since restraints are often used to keep older patients or residents from falling, an inservice that addresses this issue offers the opportunity to update the non-clinical staff on the facility's use of restraint alternatives. It will also educate the staff about the older adult's tendency to fall and correct the misconception that falls occur when restraints are not used. A second general inservice on restorative care might focus on care routines that support a restraint reduction program, reinforcing this approach as the facility's philosophy of care. Tables 3.2 and 3.3 provide sample outlines for inservices on preventing falls and providing restorative care.

RESIDENT EDUCATION

Like staff, residents may feel anxious about the change in restraint procedures. Education can help reduce or eliminate this anxiety. Often, education is geared toward residents with the highest level of cognitive function, but these people are rarely restrained for that very reason. Nevertheless, such residents may worry about how removing the restraint of other residents will affect them. Common concerns include the possibility of confused residents wandering into their rooms or the upsetting experience of seeing others fall.

Education sessions may be conducted at resident council meetings, with follow-up at unit meetings. The social services department and the nursing department can work together in addressing residents' concerns. Like staff, residents need to understand why restraints were used in the past and why this change is being attempted now. Without going into detail, a discussion of restraint alternatives is helpful. Such a discussion may focus on alternatives

Table 3.2. Sample outline for general inservice on preventing falls

I. Introduction
   A. Reasons older people may fall
      1. Normal and expected bodily changes
      2. Age-related response to illness
      3. Fear of falling that causes inactivity and further increases risk of falling
   B. Reasons falls affect everyone
      1. Resident safety is everyone's concern
      2. Everyone's increased risk of falling as a result of aging
II. Normal aging changes that put older adults at risk for falls
   A. Posture
      1. Stooped
      2. Flexed
      3. Loss of flexibility
      4. Changes in muscle mass
      5. Poor integration of various body systems
   B. Gait
      1. Decreased step height
      2. Change in base of support
      3. Poor righting reflexes
      4. Slower, stiffer walking
      5. Increased energy output, fatigue factor
   C. Vision
      1. Decreased tolerance for glare
      2. Poor visual acuity
      3. Decreased peripheral vision
      4. Poor accommodation to changing from light to darkness
      5. Increased incidence of visual pathologies
III. Other risk factors not related to the aging process
   A. Change in mental status
   B. Relocation stress
   C. Medications
   D. Underlying pathology/infection
   E. Elimination needs
IV. Decreasing the risk of falls
   A. Assessment of the resident
      1. Ability to come to standing position independently
      2. Ability to get into and out of bed
      3. Ability to move around room
      4. Ability to get on and off toilet
   B. Environmental changes to increase safety
      1. Improved lighting
      2. Lowered bed height, padded mats on floor around bed for nonambulatory residents
      3. Nonslip strips next to bed, in front of toilet
      4. Alarms
      5. Appropriate seating

(continued)

Table 3.2. (continued)

C. Nursing interventions to improve safety
   1. Observation
   2. Supervised walking
   3. Special attention to new residents
   4. Toileting schedules
V. Conclusion
   A. Occurrence of some falls despite all precautions
   B. Assessment of risk factors and intervention before a fall occurs
   C. Planning of interventions based on assessment of both the environment and the resident
   D. Fall prevention is everyone's concern

that will help residents avoid falling and procedures that will discourage confused residents from wandering into others' rooms. In time, the social services department may want to help encourage residents to be more tolerant of those who are confused and wander, but these initial meetings are probably not the best time to introduce this topic. Follow-up educational sessions should be conducted once the residents have experienced the effects of restraint removal.

FAMILY EDUCATION

Family education is best approached with both written and verbal communication. Written communication is started at the time of the resident's admission, with the admission information packet. Many residents are admitted from hospitals, where they may have been restrained. The family may think that restraints represent the only means of ensuring that the resident does not fall. Therefore, the admission material for families must include a statement of the facility's philosophy on the use of restraints. This allows families to make an informed decision about whether or not they want their relative in a facility where restraints are not the norm. In making this decision, families also need to understand the risks of routine restraint use, the benefit to the resident to be in the least restrictive environment possible, and the federal regulations stipulating that restraints not to used routinely. Most importantly, families need to know that there is no evidence that restraints prevent falls or that their removal causes them (Powell, Mitchell-Pedersen, Fingerote, & Edmund, 1989).

If the family believes strongly in the use of restraints, it is helpful for the restraint reduction program coordinator to meet with them. After admission, a conference with the family and resident is

Table 3.3. Sample outline for general inservice on providing restorative care

I. Definition of restorative care
   A. Elements on which to base individualized care
   B. Interdisciplinary care planning
      1. Improving and maintaining functional ability
      2. Fostering each individual's level of independence
II. Benefits of restorative care
   A. Benefits to the individual
      1. Increased level of function
      2. Better health
      3. Less dependence on staff for activities of daily living
      4. Greater safety
   B. Benefits to staff
      1. Division of responsibility among disciplines
      2. Improvement in communication among disciplines, using illustrative example of improving a patient's walking ability
         a. Activities department involvement
            i. Starting an exercise program to build balance and leg strength
            ii. Having patient walk rather than use wheelchair to get to activities
         b. Nursing involvement
            i. Starting a unit walking program
            ii. Helping patient or resident walk to toilet and dining room
         c. Physical therapy involvement
            i. Consulting for leg strengthening and gait training programs
            ii. Helping team set realistic goals for walking
         d. Social services involvement
            i. Communicating care plan to family
            ii. Encouraging family to help patient or resident walk during visits
            iii. Having patient or resident walk outdoors for meetings
         e. Maintenance/environmental services involvement
            i. Installing nonslip flooring
            ii. Rearranging room for safe, independent ambulation
III. Restraint removal and restorative care
   A. How restraints encourage dependence
   B. How restorative care encourages independence
IV. Individualized care
   A. Definition—care that is based on the resident's need rather than the unit's or facility's schedule
   B. Examples
      1. Addressing problem behaviors by searching for underlying cause
      2. Meeting physiological needs by implementing approaches based on individual's needs
      3. Changing environment as needed for resident's safety, comfort, and pleasure
   C. Developing care plan based on knowledge of resident and his or her life-long habits

beneficial. A postadmission care conference should focus on the needs of the resident and how, through a multidisciplinary care plan, the team hopes to meet those needs. If restraint use was an issue either before or after admission, this is an excellent opportunity to discuss alternative measures to maintain the resident's safety and autonomy. Families may be less likely to hold the facility responsible for a fall if they understand that the issue of safety was not ignored and that steps were taken to prevent a fall from occurring.

Families of previously restrained residents may have different concerns from families of newly admitted residents. It may be difficult for them to understand why restraints were necessary in the past but are no longer being used. This may be particularly difficult if the family was strongly encouraged to use restraints in the past and was reluctant to do so. Family group meetings and a family newsletter are excellent means of introducing family members to the concept of restraint reduction.

It is critical to involve families in care-planning discussions when the team is considering removing restraints. As the team develops a care plan, the family needs to be involved in discussions about restraints and alternatives. Social services and nursing can collaborate to help the family work through its discomfort with this concept. It is helpful for the family to know exactly what alternatives are being suggested and how the team thinks these will help their relatives.

Whether the resident has been restrained or not, all families should be given general information on the use of restraints. Families will want to know what the facility will do to protect residents from falls. They often find it useful to hear about specific alternatives that have been successful with other residents. Families need help to understand that older adults are likely to fall because of normal aging changes, and that although the facility will make every attempt to prevent falls, they cannot guarantee that falls will not occur. A discussion of the difficulty in balancing quality of life with safety needs may also be appropriate.

PHYSICIAN EDUCATION

The need for intervention to control problems such as falls, wandering, and agitation is usually identified by nursing staff, families, or others who are in frequent, direct contact with the resident. In the past this need has been made known to the physician in the form of a request or suggestion to order physical restraints or, in the case of agitation, to prescribe psychotropic drugs to "calm the person down." If facilities are to be successful in reducing the use of restraints, the physician must be educated about the benefits of restraint reduction and must support the use of alternative approaches. It is desirable to include the physician as a member of the team and to count him or her as an advocate for, rather than a reluctant participant in, the restraint reduction program.

The goal of educating the physician is to encourage his or her active participation in identifying alternative approaches to solving problems. Diagnosis of physical conditions that underlie the problems often suggests alternative solutions. When informed that the person has fallen several times, the physician will look for treatable medical reasons for the falls, such as low blood pressure upon standing, visual disability, anemia, and cardiac arrhythmias. An agitated resident will be evaluated for causes such as delirium, pain, or psychosis. Psychological or psychiatric evaluation will be performed after physical conditions have been ruled out. When the resident's family tells the physician that they think the person should be restrained, the physician should be the one who suggests that restraints frequently are not appropriate and that alternative approaches must be explored.

For facilities with a small number of attending physicians who visit frequently, the ideal approach is to involve the physicians and the medical director in the program from the beginning, including during the development of policies and procedures and the implementation of the in-service education program for staff. The medical director can help to identify members of the medical community who will be useful in evaluating residents and in monitoring their treatment. This may include specialists with expertise that frequently is not available to long-term care facility residents, such as psychopharmacology and pain management.

The education process must be very different for facilities with many attending physicians. The fact that most facilities do not have an organized medical staff with regular meetings makes it more difficult to reach the 50–100 physicians who see patients in the facility each year. In this situation, the medical director should encourage the education of primary care physicians throughout the community, since any of them might care for a person in the facility. Although the most effective approach varies across facilities and communities, the following suggested steps should be considered:

1. The medical director and one or more of the physicians who regularly care for residents in the facility should be involved in the development of the program. The research on the risks and bene-

fits of restraint use should be shared with them, and they should be encouraged to attend continuing medical education sessions on topics related to the care of older adults, such as falls, wandering, agitation, and depression.

2. The facility's staff, with the assistance of the medical director or other knowledgeable medical staff, should identify medical professionals in the community who may be needed for the difficult cases. Such people may include physicians with expertise in behavioral management, psychopharmacology, pain management, gait disorders, and the like, depending on the facility's resources.

3. The medical director should identify ways of reaching other physicians in the community who care for residents in the facility. Depending on the size and resources of the medical community, this may take place via a direct mailing, hospital medical staff meetings, local medical society committees and publications, or other means.

4. The medical director should contact his or her counterparts at other long-term care facilities in the neighboring area. The director should contact the directors of medical education at local hospitals and suggest continuing medical education conferences on the use of restraints and other topics related to care of older adults, such as evaluation of those who fall, common psychiatric problems, management of dementia, and the like.

5. Each time a new physician admits a person to the facility, the physician should be given information on the facility's policies and procedures regarding the use of restraints, as well as routine information on the responsibilities of the attending physician.

6. If the admitting orders for a new resident call for the use of physical or chemical restraints that are not in accord with the facility's policy and procedures, the attending physician should be notified that he or she must discuss the case with the medical director or his or her surrogate. Allowing the orders to stand until the next routine physician visit places the facility in the untenable position of not complying with its own policies and procedures.

7. The long-term care facility's staff must be assured that the medical director is available at all times to discuss difficult situations with them, the attending physician, and the family if necessary.

BOARD EDUCATION

The cooperation of the facility's governing body, whether an individual owner or a board of directors, is critical to the success of a restorative care program. The facility's philosophy and mission, as established by the board, must include a commitment to helping residents remain as independent as possible. The day-to-day operations of the facility must support this restorative care philosophy. A restorative care approach will succeed only if staff are provided with the education, administrative support, and resources to put the philosophy into practice.

Frequently, board members are lawyers, administrators, and other business people who may or may not be familiar with the clinical aspects of caring for older adults. In order to propose, develop, and support a restorative care philosophy, they must be educated about restorative care and its implications. Some central concepts to be incorporated into board education include:

1. The benefits of restorative care in terms of enhanced function and well-being of patients and residents
2. The clinical activities involved in restorative care, such as walking programs and environmental management
3. The resources, both human and material, necessary to implement a restorative care philosophy

The movement toward restraint-free care may be relatively new to many board members. They may or may not have been familiar with restraints in the first place. However, most board members are accustomed to receiving some feedback from family members about the quality of care in the facility. Hence, it is important that all board members understand the facility's restorative care approach and restraint reduction program so that they can discuss and explain these programs to family members who express concerns. Family members often question the facility's actions. (Why wasn't mother restrained so that she wouldn't fall? Why doesn't someone dress father when it's obviously so difficult for him to do so himself?) Explaining the facility's approach to care can help gain the confidence of family members and allay their fears that their relative is not being cared for properly.

Board education may include sending board members pertinent articles on other restraint removal programs and related research. Clinical staff may present a session at a regular board meeting on implementing a restorative care philosophy and a restraint removal program. This session might include an opportunity for a hands-on experience with different types of restraints and restraint alternatives. Some educators recommend demonstrating the use of restraints on volunteers from the audience during this type of experiential session. The facility needs to know its board members well to decide whether this type of experiential learning would be helpful or not. However, being able to see, touch, and manipulate wheelchair adaptations, alarms, and other restraint alternatives firsthand can enhance learning.

Board education, like staff education, should be an ongoing effort. Board members should be updated regularly on the progress of the program and the outcomes for residents, families, and staff. Such involvement and education encourages the board's support for ensuring that the facility has the resources to carry out a restorative care philosophy.

EDUCATION IN THE HOSPITAL

In the long-term care setting, education for a restraint reduction program, tends to be facility wide. In the hospital, however, education should be unit based because the needs of patients vary so much from one unit to another. For instance, using restraints on an intensive care unit to prevent a patient from pulling out a tracheostomy tube is very different from using restraints on a medical unit to prevent a patient from wandering out of his or her room.

In the hospital setting, education of staff should focus on increasing the staff's knowledge of the older person's response to illness. This will help the staff to recognize the underlying problem that is causing the behavior. Once the staff understand why the underlying behavior is occurring they can begin to look at interventions that address the problem.

Restraints should never be used as a first-line intervention. Staff in hospitals need to see restraint use only as a last resort, when all else has failed. Chapter 8 provides an excellent description of the use of restraints in the hospital setting, and is a good resource for setting up a restraint reduction program in the hospital.

CONCLUSION

The watchword in educating staff, residents, and families about restraint reduction is "be prepared." If the facility does its homework and is ready to handle questions and concerns, most situations are easily handled. Physicians and families are usually ready to comply with a restraint reduction approach once they are convinced that the staff knows how to use alternative approaches. If staff members are confident and well prepared, they will encounter much less resistance.

REFERENCES

Chang, B. (1981). Discussion. *Journal of Gerontological Nursing, 7*(10), 620–621.
Kanter, R. (1985). Managing the human side of change. *Management Review, 174*(4), 52–55.
National Citizen's Coalition for Nursing Home Reform. (1989). Handout. Washington, DC.
Powell, C., Mitchell-Pedersen, L., Fingerote, E., & Edmund, L. (1989). Freedom from restraint: Consequences of reducing physical restraints in the management of the elderly. *Canadian Medical Association Journal, 141*, 561–564.

Sample Handout for General Inservice on Removing Physical Restraints

Reducing the Use of Physical Restraints

♦ Resident Assessment

Assessment of the resident is done by the interdisciplinary team, including the nursing, medical, dietary, social work, physical therapy, occupational therapy, speech therapy, and activities departments, to identify functional ability, physical and mental status, communication skills, and interests. Assessment is continuous and ongoing.

♦ Individualized Care Plan

Each resident's care plan is based on strengths and deficits identified by assessment. The care plan must meet *individualized* resident needs and must change as the resident's needs change.

♦ Definition of Physical Restraints

Any manual method or physical or mechanical device, material, or equipment attached or adjacent to the resident's body that the resident cannot remove easily and that restricts the person's freedom of movement or normal access to his or her own body. Physical restraints and protective devices include, but are not limited to, hand mitts, soft vests and posture vests, wrist ties, wheelchair safety belts, lap trays, and toe loops.

♦ Ethical Issues

Each resident has the right to be free of physical restraint and to have his or her autonomy preserved.

♦ Negative Outcomes of Restraint Use
Changes in body systems:

Sluggish blood flow	Pressure sores
Cardiovascular stress	Decreased appetite
Chronic constipation	Increased risk of pneumonia
Incontinence	Increased risk of urinary tract
Muscle weakness	infection
Weakened bone structure	

Changes in quality of life:

Reduced social contact

Withdrawal from surroundings

Reduced participation in activities

Loss of independent or assisted mobility

Loss of independent or assisted toileting

Loss of independent or assisted bathing/dressing

Decreased desire to eat

Increased problems with sleep patterns

Increased agitation and/or depression

♦ Positive Outcomes of Restraint Use
In rare instances a restraint may enable a resident to do more than if he or she were not restrained—for example, a half-siderail may allow a partially paralyzed person to turn over. In other cases, a waist restraint may help a person whose legs have been amputated to remember that he or she cannot walk.

Alternatives to Restraint Use
General measures for avoiding use of restraints

- Provide companionship and supervision, including the use of volunteers, family, friends, and others.
- Provide physical and diversionary activity such as exercise, outdoor time, and activities that resident enjoys.
- Implement psychosocial interventions, such as following the resident's life-long habits and patterns of daily activity.
- Implement environmental approaches, such as alarms, adequate lighting, reduction of glare, individualized seating, nonslip strips, and well-placed furniture.

- Meet resident's physical needs, such as hunger, use of toilet, sleep, thirst, and exercise according to individual routine rather than facility routine.
- Train staff to meet individualized needs.

Specific measures for reducing the use of restraints

- Implement restorative care program, including walking, bowel and bladder management, independent eating, dressing, and bathing programs.
- Implement wheelchair management program to ensure that the correct chair size is used and that the chair's condition remains intact.
- Individualize facility seating for residents who do not need wheelchairs. Chairs should be tailored to meet individual needs.
- Implement specialized programs for residents with dementia to improve their quality of life.
- Increase outdoor activities.
- Implement a program that allows safe wandering while preserving others' right to privacy.
- Calm aggressive behaviors, using methods based on caregivers' knowledge of the resident.
- Prevent triggering of aggression.
- Ensure that every resident's schedule has some structure each day.

Implementation of restraint reduction program

- Be flexible in use of staff, including permanent staff assignments.
- Remove restraints on a unit-by-unit basis, one restraint at a time.
- Remove restraints in least complicated cases first.

No one person or discipline has all the answers. Success depends on the involvement of all staff members.

Adapted from National Citizen's Coalition for Nursing Home Reform, Washington, DC (1989).

Sample Handout for Follow-Up Inservice on Restraint Removal

Assessment for Restraint Removal

Assessment is the key to finding appropriate alternatives for restraints. When considering restraint use or restraint removal, the caregiver must evaluate the underlying cause of the presenting symptom, not simply the symptom itself. In long-term care facilities, restraints are often applied to prevent falls. Therefore, an assessment that evaluates residents' risk of falling is most likely to help the caregiver find the most suitable restraint alternatives. The assessment should:

I. Examine falls within the resident's environment, noting:
   A. Time of day
   B. Place
   C. Precipitating events
II. Assess the individual, noting:
   A. Gait and balance
   B. Psychosocial factors
      1. Recent admission/relocation stress
      2. Agitation
      3. Mental status
   C. Physiological factors
      1. History of falls
      2. Medications
      3. Elimination needs
      4. Visual impairments
      5. Low blood pressure upon standing
      6. Infection/pain

Restorative Care

Alternatives to restraint use are selected that improve and maintain functional ability by fostering each individual's independence and maximizing his or her level of functioning. Restorative care is based on:

- Individual assessment
- Interdisciplinary care planning
- Patient/resident centered care

Alternatives to Restraints

Alternatives to physical restraints may be placed into five categories. A restorative care plan often includes restraint alternatives from more than one category.

♦ Environmental

Wedge chair

Alternative seating

Mattress on floor next to bed at night

Nonslip strips next to bed/in bathroom

Mobility aids

Body props

Antitippers on wheelchairs

Visual barriers (camouflage) for doors

Decreased/increased light; night-light

Beds with wheels removed; lowered beds

Beds without siderails

Alarm system

♦ Activities

Structured activities

Television, radio, music

Something to hold (e.g., towel, blanket)

Fine motor apron with attached zippers, fabric swatches, etc.

Exercise

Social activity

Training in activities of daily living

◆ Psychosocial

Companionship
Therapeutic touching
Active listening
Behavior modification
Remotivation
Reality orientation
Quiet time

◆ Physiological

Pain relief
Change in treatment (e.g., remove intravenous lines, catheters)
Physical or occupational therapy
Correction of dehydration, treatment of infection
Sensory aids
Assessment of all medications

◆ Nursing Care Routines

Daily walking schedule
Toileting schedules
Supervision of activities of daily living
Observation of resident (relocate person near nurses' station)
Frequent reminders to resident not to get up without help
Tracking of wanderers every half hour
Attention to residents' comfort needs
Attention to residents' physical positioning
Addition or removal of drugs
Napping
Alternatives to use in case of nighttime awakening:
    Toileting
    Snack provision
    Reassessment of comfort level
    Relocation next to nurses' station
    Placement in recliner chair instead of bed
    Permission to remain awake if resident is not sleepy

Chapter 4

Implementing a Restraint Removal Program

Vivian J. Koroknay

Even after the staff members and the patients' or residents' families have been prepared for restraint removal (see Chapters 2 and 3), the road to reduced restraint use may still be rocky. Change is always difficult, and removing restraints involves changing a once-acceptable standard of care. Intellectually, staff, families, and physicians may understand why the use of restraints should be discontinued, but emotionally they may feel insecure and anxious about this process. Ongoing administrative support, education, and one-to-one interventions are essential once the process of restraint removal is actually underway.

THE RESTRAINT REMOVAL PROCESS

Restraint removal is best carried out one unit at a time, and one patient or resident at a time. Removing restraints one by one allows the staff's confidence to build with each success. Progressing unit by unit also allows the units to build on each others' successes. By the time one unit has removed all, or almost all, of its restraints, other units will hear that it can be done and will be more receptive to beginning the process.

When selecting the unit on which the restraint removal program will begin, it is best to select a unit on which the transition will most likely be smooth and the program successful. A unit whose nurse manager is open to new ideas and expresses at least some support for the program is probably a good choice. It is helpful, too, if this unit has not relied too strongly on restraints in the past.

Once the unit has been chosen, meetings with all three shifts should be arranged. The social worker, activities coordinator, and dietitian or dietary aide assigned to the unit should be included at these meetings. Chapter 3 examines in detail the educational process that should occur at these meetings. At the very least, the following steps should be included:

1. Review the restraint removal policy and procedure thoroughly.

2. Discuss the process by which restraints will be removed to make sure that staff members understand clearly that restraints will be removed one at a time and that each patient or resident will be assessed and observed before the restraint order is discontinued.

3. Remind staff that all patients or residents will be considered for restraint removal.

4. Call for feedback from staff to determine whose restraints will be the easiest to remove and whose should be removed first.

5. Discuss possible alternatives, such as what has worked before with patients or residents on other units and what is likely to work well with the patients or residents on the present unit.

When deciding whose restraint to remove first, staff should assess each patient's or resident's risk of falling (see Chapter 5). For instance, if the person is wheelchair-bound, the risk of falling from the chair must be considered. Anyone will try to get out of a chair if he or she is uncomfortable, but a nonambulatory resident will fall if that attempt is made. Therefore, the individual's sitting posture and the fit of the chair need to be considered when assessing the patient or resident for risk of falling. The assessment may also indicate whether medications should be adjusted to help ensure safety. All possible fall hazards should be addressed before the patient or resident is observed without a restraint. Once the assessment has been completed and changes have been made to ensure safety, the restraint removal process may begin.

Before an order for restraints is discontinued, it is important for the restraint removal coordinator to observe the patient or resident without a restraint. This helps reassure the staff that restraints are being removed cautiously. It is best to observe the patient or resident without the restraint at times when he or she is most likely to be active. The late morning period before lunch or the late afternoon usually are times when the coordinator can get a fairly realistic impression of the person's most active behavior. The observation period may last a few days. Although the restraint removal coordinator conducts this first observation, after a while staff may be made responsible for observing the patient or resident. During this "trial" time, it is a good idea to place the untied restraint across the back of the person's wheelchair. This alerts all staff members that the person is being observed for restraint removal. It also reassures the nursing staff that if the person grows restless and the staff believe that he or she is not safe without the restraint, it can be reapplied temporarily, until the restraint removal coordinator can reassess the person. In fact, staff rarely put the person's restraint back on. However, in the beginning, it is reassuring for the staff to know they may do so if necessary.

As the removal process continues with other patients or residents, the coordinator can continue to observe those people whose restraints already have been removed. This gives the coordinator a chance to evaluate the success of the suggested interventions and to make changes in the care plan as needed. Because patients' or residents' needs change frequently due to illness or improved health, the restraint removal care plan must be dynamic. It, too, must change along with the individual. However, the restraint removal process itself should not change significantly. It should always include the following steps:

1. Assess the patient's or resident's risk of falling.
2. Minimize that risk by implementing preventative interventions.
3. Untie the restraint.
4. Observe the person without the restraint.
5. Make adjustments in the care plan.
6. Discontinue the restraint.

It is best not to set a deadline by which the unit must be restraint free. Staff members will indicate what they are capable of handling and it is best to proceed at the pace they set. Often, the nursing staff will have begun to experiment with removing a person's restraint for brief periods even before the restraint removal coordinator assesses that person. This is a strong indication that staff members are beginning to feel comfortable with the concept and that the process can proceed a little more quickly.

THE INTERDISCIPLINARY CARE PLAN

The care plan is pivotal to the success of the restraint removal process. The process should involve many disciplines, and the care plan itself should reflect this. A typical restraint removal care plan for an ambulatory patient or resident might include environmental alternatives, physiological alternatives, activities, and nursing care interventions, as described in Chapter 5. An example might be a resident who has advanced Parkinson's disease and is still ambulatory, but falls frequently and hence is unsafe. After performing an assessment, the care team makes a list of alternatives to help avoid having to use a restraint (see Table 4.1).

There is a tendency to view restraint use as a nursing problem, or to believe that one department can provide all of the necessary interventions. This is not the case. A multidisciplinary approach is crucial to the success of a restraint removal program. Safe restraint removal is a facility-wide endeavor. The administration's support of an approach that involves interdisciplinary cooperation and problem solving is central to the success of a restraint reduction program.

Although the interdisciplinary approach to restraint reduction is vital, the role of the nursing assistant cannot be overlooked. Nursing assistants provide most of the direct care in nursing homes. Therefore, any change in how care is given must consider the role of the nursing assistant. Change in resident or patient care will not take place unless the nursing assistants are provided with the education and support they need to accept that change.

Since nursing assistants give the direct care to the patients or residents, they, more than anyone else on the caregiving team, know the resident's actions and habits. If falls are a concern in removing a restraint, the nursing assistant is likely to know when the resident is most restless and hence when the resident is most likely to fall. Having this input in developing the care plan will increase the likelihood of its success. Even if the nursing assistant is unable to provide this information, he or she still needs to be a part of the care plan's development since the nursing assistant will be providing, or assisting others to provide, many of the restraint alternatives.

Often, nursing assistants other than the primary nursing assistants are involved in giving the direct care. It is important that these individuals know what is expected of them with respect to restraint reduction. In addition to verbal communication via the shift-to-shift report, it is helpful to provide written communication. One way of doing this is to place instructions in the resident's room. Placing restraint reduction instructions on the same color paper throughout the facility provides a visual cue to everyone entering the room that the resident has a restraint reduction care plan in effect. Fluorescent papers can be particularly helpful in calling attention to the instructions. Placing brief instructions in the residents' rooms enables any nursing assistant who is caring for the resident to follow the restraint reduction care plan. This is an essential component of providing continuity of care.

Table 4.1. Sample interdisciplinary care plan for an older adult with Parkinson's disease

Intervention	Desired result	Department
Environmental		
Place nonslip strips next to bed, in front of toilet	Safer footing going to the bathroom	Engineering, environmental services
Remove wheels from bed	Safer exit from bed	Engineering, environmental services
Activity-related		
Encourage attendance at afternoon activities	Diversion when nursing staff are unavailable	Activities, volunteer
Encourage taking morning walks, supervised by volunteer, outdoors if possible	Exercise to help maintain ability to walk and strengthen lower extremities; diversionary activity	Volunteer, nursing
Physiological		
Adjust dosage of sinemet	Improved control of Parkinson's symptoms	Medicine, nursing
Set up physical therapy consult	Gait analysis; assessment of need to switch from cane to walker	Physical therapy
Nursing care		
Initiate toileting schedule	Fewer falls in bathroom; improved continence	Nursing
Evaluate care plan	Understanding of success in terms of fewer falls, improved mental outlook, improved functional gait	All departments

COMMON PROBLEMS IN IMPLEMENTING A RESTRAINT REMOVAL PROGRAM

Changing an acceptable standard of care can be difficult. Staff may often believe that restraints are the only option. During the initial staff meetings at which restraint removal is discussed, nursing assistants often claim that they cannot remove restraints because residents will fall. At this early stage of planning, it is important to make sure that all staff realize that every patient or resident will be considered for restraint removal. Often, it is helpful to discuss some of the various alternatives that have worked for other patients or residents. Staff members also need to understand that long-term care facilities cannot guarantee absolute safety for their residents. Therefore, if the nursing staff follow the restraint removal care plan and the resident falls, that resident will be reassessed, but the staff will not be held responsible for the fall. If, however, staff fail to follow the care plan and a resident falls, then the incident will be investigated.

Often, staff members may be reluctant to carry out some of the nursing interventions necessary in restraint removal, or simply "forget" to do so. For instance, the staff may not understand how toilet schedules fit into the restraint removal program. It is essential that everyone—nursing staff, physicians, families, and the residents or patients themselves—understand the purpose of each intervention. Understanding improves compliance and may help staff members find alternatives for other patients or residents.

Families and physicians often voice concern about and even resistance to discontinuing restraints. They may be unwilling to risk that the patient or resident may fall. Although physicians may be aware of the OBRA regulations, they still need additional education and reassurance. The attending physician should be told what interventions the staff members will implement to protect the patient or resident and thus decrease the physician's potential liability for falls. Simply asking the physician to change the restraint order without discussing the new care plan will not be enough.

Some of the family's concerns may be addressed by involving them in designing the interdisciplinary care plan. Family members are more likely to accept the plan if they feel that they are consulted and are encouraged to contribute. Implementing the program's later stages will also be easier if physicians and family members are introduced to the concept of restraint removal in the early stages of policy development.

Sometimes, even after consultation and education have been provided, a physician or a family is adamant that a restraint not be removed. All facilities should have a plan for dealing with such resistance. Such a plan can include the following:

1. Refer the family and/or physician to the facility's medical director or administrator for further discussion.

2. Obtain a documented statement of informed consent, signed by an authorized individual requesting the restraint be used.

3. Review restraint use and informed consent on a regular basis, as often as once a week, depending on the facility's policy and procedure regarding use.

After the restraint reduction program has been implemented on all the units, there may still be situations where staff may revert to using restraints. In periods of stress, for instance, when there is low staffing or high acuity, it is not uncommon for staff members to resume old habits. Even if staff do not actually revert to using a restraint, they may need to call on the restraint reduction coordinator if they are unable to formulate a care plan that utilizes restraint alternatives when faced with a difficult patient or resident problem. It is important that the restraint reduction coordinator maintain this role even a year after the restraint reduction program is implemented. Some staff may still have not internalized the change in philosophy regarding restraint use and may thus require ongoing assistance to address issues such as falls and wandering that in the past were resolved by using restraints.

There are a number of ways that the restraint coordinator can ensure that restraint use does not once again become a first choice in solving patient or resident care problems. One way to avoid this "back slide" is to analyze falls and behavior problems within the facility. This can be done by monitoring the incident reports. Once the restraint reduction coordinator recognizes a "frequent faller" or a resident with episodes of wandering or other behavior problems from the incident reports, steps can be taken to address the situation. Intervening with problem-solving techniques at the early stages of the problem is more likely to produce restraint alternatives than will intervening after the restraint has already been considered or already applied. Monitoring falls will also reassure unit staff that there has not been an increase in falls since restraints have been removed. This is important information for maintaining staff members' confidence in the restraint reduction program.

When staff members are not completely at ease with the philosophy of restraint-free care, they are unlikely to draw on past successes with restraint removal. Instead, each time a problem arises where a restraint could be considered, staff may be at a loss to develop alternatives. The restraint removal coordinator needs to be available to the staff to assist them to draw on their past successes and to facilitate the development of a care plan that does not include the use of a restraint. Without the restraint removal coordinator to continue these interventions with the staff, restraints may very well return to the facility in force.

The implementation phase is difficult at times because everyone who is involved in caring for a patient or resident must change his or her basic philosophy about health care for older people. Some resistance to the restraint removal program can and should be expected. Educating and reassuring staff, families, and physicians, and involving them in the planning and implementation process will help ensure the program's ultimate success.

Part II

Reducing the Use of Physical Restraints

Chapter 5

Assessment for Physical Restraint Removal

Vivian J. Koroknay and Patricia Carter

Assessment is the first step in considering restraint removal. Behaviors that often result in restraint use, such as falling, wandering, and agitation, have an underlying cause, and an assessment of the patient or resident is necessary to identify that cause. Although a formal assessment tool may or may not be necessary, some form of assessment is needed to make a systematic selection from the appropriate restraint alternatives. This chapter examines factors that should be assessed when considering patients or residents for restraint removal or restraint application. In particular, factors that increase the risk of falling are examined.

The assessment process begins by determining why a restraint was applied in the first place or why a restraint is now being considered. Often, staff members feel compelled to use physical restraints when a patient or resident falls, wanders, or is agitated. The reason for using or considering using the restraint will affect the assessment and the alternatives selected. To determine why a restraint is being used, staff should ask the following questions:

For falls:

1. What time of day does the patient or resident fall?
2. Where do the falls occur?
3. What is the person doing when he or she falls? (Determine the precipitating event, such as climbing into bed at night.)

For wandering:

1. When does the patient or resident wander?
2. Where is the person's destination? Outside of the building, or within the confines of the unit?
3. What problems does the wandering cause? Can the person be allowed to wander at will?

For agitation:

1. At what time of day does the patient or resident tend to become agitated?
2. Does a certain event precipitate the agitation?

Answering these questions before performing a complete assessment can be helpful and may save time in the long run. For instance, if the patient or resident frequently falls while getting into bed at night, the bed may be too high and may need to be lowered by having the wheels removed. If the person tends to become agitated late in the afternoon and tries to get out of the wheelchair, then the best intervention may be to have him or her take a nap after lunch. Usually, however, the solutions to problems are not this evident, and a more complete assessment must be done. Additional information on assessment for chemical restraint reduction appears in Chapter 13.

Often, the decision to restrain is based on the need to prevent the patient or resident from falling (Cutchins, 1991; Frengley & Mion 1986; Sloane et al., 1991; Strumpf & Evans, 1988). Indeed, once a person has fallen, a restraint is often used regardless of the outcome of the fall (Evans & Strumpf, 1989). Therefore, a restraint removal assessment should focus on factors that may increase the risk of falling. Identifying patients or residents who are at risk for falling allows the staff to intercede and thus prevent falls before they occur. This, in turn, decreases the need for restraints.

An assessment should address factors that affect gait and balance, as well as other variables that can cause falls. A tool developed by Berryman, Gaskin, Jones, Tolley, and MacMullen (1989) addresses many of the factors that place older adults at risk for falls, but it is not specific to the long-term care facility setting. The following sections describe these factors as well as other physiological and psychological factors that are specific to the long-term care setting.

GAIT AND BALANCE

Walking is a primary functional task whose goal is to get a person from point A to point B. Gait difficulty or deviation directly affects one's ability to function normally. For this reason, the performance,

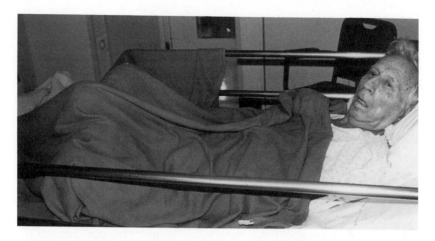

Prolonged immobilization of the older person can have many negative effects on physiological functions and will eventually place the person at increased risk for falls. (Photograph courtesy of the Hebrew Home of Greater Washington. Used by permission.)

or functionally oriented, gait evaluation is a quick way for the professional staff to assess a person's gait and ability to walk safely or with minimal risk (Glickstein, 1991). Gait assessment is best performed by observing the person performing his or her daily routines, such as walking in the hall, sitting on and rising from the toilet, and getting into and out of bed. Discussing the ability to carry on the activities of daily living with the nursing assistant will augment the evaluation process.

Specifically, all assessments of gait should examine the following:

1. *Difficulty rising and sitting back down.* The sit-to-stand motion is often referred to as the "gateway to independence" (Kaufman, 1988, p. 18). This motion requires the body's center of mass to move forward and upward, and to recover from the movement. It requires normal strength, range of motion, coordination, and balance control, and hence is an accurate initial indicator of the patient's or resident's functional ability.

2. *Instability when first standing.* Loss of balance control is one of the most frightening experiences for an older adult. Several factors increase the risk of balance problems and falls. Major factors are problems with blood pressure regulation, changes in the neurological system, changes in strength and flexibility, and physical obstacles in the environment. The person's ability to keep his or her balance when standing should be evaluated carefully.

3. *Need for assistance when ambulating.* Some indications of a person's ability to walk are the amount of staff assistance he or she needs and/or how much assistance the patient or resident asks for.

4. *Use of assistive devices.* A patient's or resident's need to use an assistive device, such as a walker, alerts the clinician that stability has been compromised. If the person is confused, he or she may forget to ask for assistance or forget to use the assistive device. The clinician should make sure that the ambulation aids are in good working condition, are measured to fit the resident or patient, and are used appropriately.

5. *Fit of shoes and type of shoes.* Poorly fitting shoes compromise a person's gait and safety. Patients or residents who have shoe problems may experience pain while bearing weight. Foot deformities such as corns, bunions, hammer toes, and calluses can be aggravated by poorly fitting shoes, and ambulation can be impeded as a result. Pain may cause a person to deviate from a steady gait pattern in an effort to alleviate the pain. Patients and residents should wear proper footwear, such as low-heeled, closed-toe supportive shoes.

6. *Severely decreased gait speed.* Walking speed is an important factor in gait stability. Studies have indicated that walking speed decreases with increased functional dependency. The average adult walks approximately 90–120 steps per minute. Changes in a smooth, coordinated pattern markedly reduces the person's walking efficiency and greatly increases his or her energy expenditure. Muscle weakness, pain, and fatigue can also reduce the number of steps per minute.

7. *Short, discontinuous, shuffling steps.* Subtle changes in shifts from heel to toe, from right to left foot, and from heel-strike to toe-off may indicate a potential gait instability that will increase the patient's or resident's risk of gait instability. The average length of an adult's step is approximately 15 inches. With neuromuscular changes, fatigue, or disease, the step length may decrease (Larish, Martin, & Mungiole, 1988). The width of the base of support should not exceed 2–4 inches from heel to heel. If the person is walking with a wider base of support, the clinician should suspect an underlying pathology. However, older adults often develop a wide base of support to compensate for other gait problems, such as dizziness or unsteadiness. Such factors may be caused by cerebellar problems or decreased sensation in the sole of the foot (Steinberg, 1978).

8. *Staggering when turning around.* The evaluator should be sure to notice whether the patient or resident turns his or her whole body rather than just the head to look around. When neck movement is decreased, the brain receives less information on body position. Older adults who turn their whole body may be getting too little stimulation of the nerve endings in the neck (Woolacolt, 1982).

9. *Swaying off a straight path when walking.* Some older adults walk slowly and unsteadily, and sway from side to side. They frequently use walls, chairs, and other available objects as support when walking.

10. *Changes in gait pattern when walking through a doorway.* A decrease in proprioception, or the sense of body position in space, may affect one's ability to maneuver in the environment. The patient or resident, when approaching a doorway, stair, or change in the walking surface's elevation, may become unsure and grab at the walls and/or slow his or her gait speed and shuffle.

11. *Lurching or slapping.* Muscular imbalance and/or muscle weakness in older adults contribute to unsteady gait patterns. A deviation from the smooth, symmetrical pattern of walking affects stability and can increase the risk of falling. It is important for the clinician to note any changes in the resident's or patient's gait. A change in gait may indicate onset of a new pathology or worsening of an existent pathology and may further increase the risk of falling.

For nonambulatory patients or residents, an assessment should be made of their sitting posture in a chair and/or wheelchair. Restraints are frequently used to correct improper positioning resulting from poor sitting posture. However, chairs and wheelchairs can be adapted to meet postural weaknesses so that restraints are not necessary. Chapter 6 examines normal sitting posture and seating adaptations to ensure proper alignment of the spine.

PHYSIOLOGICAL FACTORS

As people age, subtle changes take place that affect their physiological equilibrium. These changes may affect gait and balance adversely, and may cause agitation and wandering, which are common precursors to the use of restraints. To help prevent the unnecessary use of restraints, the clinician should assess the potential negative effects of each of the factors discussed in the following sections.

Change in Health Status

Delirium, falls, and incontinence frequently indicate an underlying acute illness in older adults (Irvine, 1990). Falls can occur as a result of the illness or the subsequent weakness from it, or they may be a side effect of treatment (Chenitz, Kussman, & Stone, 1991). Patients or residents who have experienced a cluster of falls should be assessed for an underlying infection.

History of Falling

Patients or residents who have fallen once are at increased risk of falling again. Research has shown that they are often restrained regardless of the consequences of the fall (Strumpf & Evans, 1988). Therefore, a history of falling is a component of the restraint removal assessment. If a person has a history of falling, determining whether a pattern exists in the time or place of the fall will help the clinician understand the cause of such falls. As an example, consider a resident who was given Serax as needed for acute anxiety. After she had fallen several times, caregivers reviewed her chart and found that her falls always occurred within 2 hours of receiving the Serax. When the drug was stopped and another antianxiety agent was selected, the falls stopped. Clearly, this resident did not need to be restrained. If her history had not been analyzed, she might have been restrained unnecessarily.

Medications

The effect of drugs on older adults cannot be overstated. Older people are at increased risk of adverse side effects from drugs for several reasons. Normal aging changes affect the pharmacokinetics and pharmacodynamics of drugs, as do changes in nutritional status. Many older adults take numerous drugs to treat several different conditions (Ebersole & Hess, 1985; Stone, 1991). Certain drugs have been implicated in causing loss of balance and falls, lethargy, and altered mental status. Since these behaviors often lead to restraint use, uncovering an adverse drug effect can help lead to restraint removal.

A good rule of thumb to follow in assessing an older adult is that "any symptom in an elderly patient may be a drug side effect until proved otherwise" (Avorn & Gurwitz, 1990, p. 71). Often, the most unexpected drug can cause problems for the older person. For instance, nonsteroidal antiinflammatory drugs (NSAIDs), heralded as an effective alternative to narcotics in pain control, have been shown to cause dizziness, confusion, and mood swings (Granek et al., 1987).

Although these drugs may still be a good choice for treating chronic pain, their use should be suspected if the patient's or resident's mental status changes or if he or she falls.

Another point to remember is that in older people, the range within which a drug is therapeutically effective tends to be very narrow. Although it is generally accepted that older adults require smaller doses of drugs than do younger people, adverse drug effects still occur even at the reduced doses. For example, consider a resident experiencing lower back pain who was started on a very small dose of Darvocet. Within a few days, the resident exhibited lethargy and a change in gait. The drug was stopped and the resident subsequently improved. In assessing patients or residents, caregivers should consider the effects of all drugs on behavior and gait.

Visual Impairment

Visual impairment is often a factor when older adults fall (Rhymes & Jaeger, 1988; Tinetti & Speechley, 1989). Loss of visual acuity and diminished ability to adapt when changing from light to dark are normal aging changes (Burrage, Dixon, & Sehy, 1991). In addition, older people are also more prone to cataracts, macular degeneration, and glaucoma (Tinetti & Speechley, 1989). Balance is maintained, in part, by input from the visual sensory system (Rhymes & Jaeger, 1988). Therefore, any disruption in this system will affect balance and increase the risk of falls. The institutional environment common to both hospitals and long-term care facilities further compounds the effects of limited vision. Long hallways and fluorescent lights increase distortion of the visual field. These conditions not only make it difficult for the person to see where he or she is going, but also obscure obstacles in the way. Diminished vision may also cause sensory deprivation and disorientation. As a result, the resident or patient may become confused or agitated when he or she cannot make sense of the environment.

Elimination

Problems with continence may lead to falls and agitation. Older adults who have urge incontinence or stress incontinence often rush to the bathroom in an attempt to prevent an "accident." This rushing may cause them to be less attentive to safe walking, possibly causing them to fall. For residents or patients who are confined to a wheelchair, sitting on a wet pad may cause them to become agitated or restless in the wheelchair. Residents who are not attended to immediately often will try to get up unassisted and are likely to fall.

Postural Hypotension

Postural hypotension is defined as a 20 mm Hg drop in the systolic blood pressure accompanied by a 10 mm Hg drop in the diastolic when the person stands up (Burrage et al., 1991). Approximately 20% of people over 65, and 30%–50% of people over 75 years of age have this condition (Robbins & Rubenstein, 1984). It is caused by various neurological disorders, dehydration, anemia, and certain medications. Among residents in long-term care facilities, it has also been found to occur after meals (Burrage et al., 1991). Often, people with postural hypotension will exhibit no symptoms.

Postural hypotension may be implicated in about 20% of falls among people over 75 (Robbins & Rubenstein, 1984). Every person should be checked at admission for postural hypotension, since it is clearly a risk factor in falls. Blood pressure should be checked while the person is lying, sitting, and standing. Residents who fall more than once should also be checked to see if postural hypotension could be the cause.

PSYCHOSOCIAL FACTORS

Recent Admission

Studies on the use of restraints have indicated that older adults often are restrained within 24 hours of admission to a facility and that the restraints are left in place until they are discharged (Mion, Frengley, Jakovcic, & Marino, 1989; Robbins, Boyko, Lane, Cooper, & Jahnigan, 1987; Strumpf & Evans, 1988). When performing the assessment for removing a person's restraints, both psychological and physical deterioration must be considered. Both are common in older adults who have experienced a change in their environment (Wells & Mac-Donald, 1981). For the older person whose health may already be impaired, relocation to a hospital or long-term care facility can be particularly stressful (Rosswurm, 1983). A 1989 study by Brooke found that 54% of older adults who were admitted to long-term care facilities suffered from fatigue, restlessness, and loss of appetite. Recent admission to such a facility has also been shown to increase residents' risk of falling and therefore is a factor that should be considered when assessing for restraint use or restraint removal (Berryman et al., 1989; Gross, Shimamoto, Rose, & Frank, 1990; Rhymes & Jaeger, 1988).

Memory/Recall Ability

An older adult's memory and ability to recall are important measures of cognitive ability that are frequently used to decide whether or not the person should be restrained. People who are restrained tend to have more serious cognitive deficits and lower functional ability than do those who are not restrained. In both long-term care facilities and hospitals, restraint use increases as both age and cognitive impairment increase (Evans & Strumpf, 1989). One reason memory and recall ability play a particularly important role in restraint use is that the resident may not remember that he or she cannot walk independently and is therefore at increased risk for falls. Another reason is that people with impaired memory are more likely to wander away from the unit or the facility because they cannot remember where they live.

"Problem Behavior"

The Minimum Data Set for Nursing Home Resident Assessment and Care Screening (MDS) defines "problem behaviors" as wandering, verbally or physically abusive behavior, or socially inappropriate disruptive behavior. These behaviors are very similar to those described in a study by Marx, Cohen-Mansfield, and Werner (1990). That study defined agitated behaviors as abusive or aggressive behavior, appropriate behavior that is performed at an inappropriate frequency, or behavior that is inappropriate for a given social situation. It found that residents of long-term care facilities who fell behaved in these ways more often that did those who did not fall (Marx et al., 1990). The increased risk of falls certainly makes these residents more likely to be restrained. Evans and Strumpf (1989) also state that agitation and behavior problems are predictors of restraint use. Evans (1987) found increased restraint use among residents who exhibited symptoms of sundown syndrome, the onset or worsening of confusion in the late afternoon or early evening hours. Therefore, the presence of problem behaviors is a factor that should be assessed when restraint removal is being considered.

CONCLUSION

Clearly, many conditions among older adults are associated with restraint use. Although the list in this chapter is not exhaustive, it gives the health care team some insight into needs that require intervention. Removing restraints means finding alternatives that work, but such alternatives can be found only after the underlying problem is uncovered. An assessment for restraint removal must consider the many factors that affect the health care provider's decision to restrain. Identifying these needs is the first step in finding appropriate alternatives to restraints.

REFERENCES

Avorn, J., & Gurwitz, J. (1990). Principles of pharmacology. In C.K. Cassel, D.E. Riesenberg, L.S. Sorensen, & J.R. Walsh (Eds.), *Geriatric medicine* (2nd ed.) (pp. 66–78). New York: Springer-Verlag.

Berryman, E., Gaskin, D., Jones, A., Tolley, F., & MacMullen, J. (1989). Point by point predicting elders' falls. *Geriatric Nursing, 10*(4), 199–201.

Brooke, V. (1989). How elders adjust. *Geriatric Nursing, 10*(2), 66–68.

Burrage, R., Dixon, L., & Sehy, Y. (1991). Physical assessment. In W.C. Chenitz, J.T. Stone, & S.A. Salisbury (Eds.), *Clinical gerontological nursing: A guide to advanced practice* (pp. 27–47). Philadelphia: W.B. Saunders.

Chenitz, C., Kussman, H., & Stone, J. (1991). Preventing falls. In W.C. Chenitz, J.T. Stone, & S.A. Salisbury (Eds.), *Clinical gerontological nursing: A guide to advanced practice* (pp. 309–324). Philadelphia: W.B. Saunders.

Cutchins, C. (1991). Blueprint for restraint free care. *American Journal of Nursing, 91*(7), 36–43.

Ebersole, P., & Hess, P. (1985). Drug use and abuse. In P. Ebersole & P. Hess (Eds.), *Toward healthy aging* (pp. 272–299). St. Louis: C.V. Mosby.

Evans, L. (1987). Sundown syndrome in institutionalized elderly. *Journal of the American Geriatrics Society, 35*(2), 101–108.

Evans, L., & Strumpf, N. (1989). Tying down the elderly: A review of the literature on physical restraints. *Journal of the American Geriatrics Society, 37*(1), 65–74.

Frengley, J., & Mion, L. (1986). Incidence of physical restraints on acute medical wards. *Journal of the American Geriatrics Society, 34*, 562–568.

Glickstein, J.K. (1991). Gait and gait training in the elderly. *Geriatric Care and Rehabilitation, 4*(10), 4.

Granek, E., Baker, S., Abbey, J., Robinson, E., Myers, A., Samkorr, J., & Klein, L. (1987). Medications and diagnoses in relation to falls in a long-term care facility. *American Geriatrics Society, 35*, 503–511.

Gross, Y., Shimamoto, Y., Rose, C., & Frank, B. (1990). Why do they fall? Monitoring risk factors in nursing homes. *Journal of Gerontological Nursing, 16*(6), 20–25.

Irvine, P. (1990). Patterns of disease: The challenge of multiple illnesses. In C.K. Cassel, D.E. Riesenberg, L.S. Sorensen, & J.R. Walsh (Eds.), *Geriatric Medicine* (2nd ed.) (pp. 96–101). New York: Springer-Verlag.

Kaufman, T. (1988). *Physical therapy for the frail elderly.* Bethesda, MD: Professional Health Education.

Larish, D., Martin, P., & Mungiole, M. (1988). Characteristic patterns of gait in the healthy old. *Annals of the New York Academy of Sciences, 515*, 18–32.

Marx, M., Cohen-Mansfield, J., & Werner, P. (1990). Agitation and falls in institutionalized elderly persons. *Journal of Applied Gerontology, 9*(1), 106–117.

Mion, L., Frengley, D., Jakovic, C., & Marino, J. (1989). A further exploration of the use of physical restraints in hospitalized patients. *Journal of the American Geriatrics Society, 37*(19), 949–956.

Rhymes, J., & Jaeger, R. (1988). Falls: Prevention and management in the institutional setting. *Clinics in Geriatric Medicine, 4*(3), 613–621.

Robbins, A., & Rubenstein, L. (1984). Postural hypotension in the elderly. *Journal of the American Geriatrics Society, 32*, 769.

Robbins, L., Boyko, E., Lane, J., Cooper, D., & Jahnigan, D. (1987). Binding the elderly: A prospective study in an acute care hospital. *Journal of the American Geriatrics Society, 35*(4), 90–296.

Rosswurm, M. (1983). Relocation and the elderly. *Journal of Gerontological Nursing, 9*(12), 632–637.

Sloane, P., Mathew, M., Scarborough, J., Desai, G., Koch, G., & Tangen, C. (1991). Physical and pharmacologic restraint of nursing home patients with dementia. *Journal of the American Medical Association, 265*(10), 1278–1282.

Steinberg, F. (1978). Gait disorders in the aged. *Journal of the American Geriatrics Society, 20*, 537–540.

Stone, J. (1991). Preventing physical iatrogenic problems. In W.C. Chenitz, J.T. Stone, & S.A. Salisbury (Eds.), *Clinical gerontological nursing: A guide to advanced practice* (pp. 359–373). Philadelphia: W.B. Saunders.

Strumpf, N., & Evans, L. (1988). Physical restraint of the hospitalized elderly: Perceptions of patients and nurses. *Nursing Research, 37*(3), 132–137.

Tinetti, M., & Speechley, M. (1989). Prevention of falls among the elderly. *New England Journal of Medicine, 320*(16), 1055–1059.

Wells, L., & MacDonald, G. (1981). Interpersonal networks and post relocation adjustment of the institutionalized elderly. *The Gerontologist, 21*(2), 177–182.

Woolacolt, M. (1982). Postural reflexes and aging. *Advances in Neurogerontology, 3*, 98–119.

Chapter 6

Environmental and Nursing Alternatives to Physical Restraints

Patricia Carter and Vivian J. Koroknay

Providing an environment for older adults that promotes their physiological and psychosocial well-being is a challenge facing all long-term care providers. The challenge begins with removing restraints. Implementing a restraint reduction program can be troublesome, because it means changing the standard of care. Until recently, restraints have been an acceptable means of protecting patients and residents who are at risk of falling or wandering. To stop using restraints means balancing safety with freedom. In short, it means taking some risks.

In finding alternatives to restraints, the emphasis is not on removing the restraints but on creating an environment in which restraints are not needed in the first place. This is part of a restorative care approach. Restorative care fosters independence and maximizes each individual's level of functioning. Focusing on individual needs, rather than unit schedules, is essential to the restorative care concept. This might mean putting off making a bed in favor of helping a patient or resident walk to the toilet so that he or she is less likely to get out of a chair unassisted and fall.

An interdisciplinary approach is central to promoting restorative care. All departments must be involved in the process of creating and maintaining the least restrictive environment possible. For example, the maintenance department can apply nonslip strips to the floors to keep older people from sliding when getting up from the toilet or the bed. The activities department can provide therapeutic exercises that decrease restlessness and strengthen muscles. Each discipline brings its area of expertise to the patient's or resident's care plan. By working together, staff can begin to remove restraints and meet individual needs.

Before alternatives to restraints can be found, it is important to assess the care needs that led to the initial use of the restraint. An individualized approach is the key. An example is the patient or resident who has poor sitting posture following a stroke. Close evaluation reveals that the person's posture deteriorates only after sitting up for 2 hours. In the restorative care approach, rather than applying a posture vest, the caregiver addresses the individual's need by allowing him or her to go back to bed for a while after sitting up for 2 hours.

When a patient or resident has been restrained for an extended period of time, it can take a bit of detective work to discover the circumstances that led to restraint use. Often, once restraints have been put on, they are left on without further evaluation. However, in the restorative care plan, ongoing evaluation and assessment are essential. (Chapter 5 presents an in-depth examination of assessment.)

The reasons for using restraints are as many and varied as the people on whom they are used. Thus, alternatives to restraints do not form neat categories from which the health care provider may choose. However, some basic categories of alternatives may be used when deciding whether to remove restraints. This chapter examines environmental and activities-related alternatives to restraints as well as physiological and nursing care alternatives.

ENVIRONMENTAL CHANGES AS AN ALTERNATIVE TO RESTRAINTS

The physical environment can play an integral part in a patient's or resident's ability to function independently and safely. Often, minor changes can make the difference between being restrained and being free. Assessment for restraint removal should address whether or not the person's falls follow a pattern. Caregivers should determine:

1. Where the patient or resident falls
2. When the patient or resident falls
3. Whether a precipitating factor seems to be common to most of the falls (e.g., falling while trying to get to the toilet)

The answers to these questions will alert the staff to any safety hazards in the immediate environment.

In assessing the environment for safety, it is important to watch the patient or resident functioning in his or her immediate surroundings. Three key areas to note are the person's ability to:

1. Maneuver in his or her room
2. Get into and out of bed
3. Get on and off the toilet

The sections that follow examine these three components of the assessment process and changes in the environment that can help ensure greater safety for patients and residents.

Furniture Arrangement

Even if the patient's or resident's falls do not follow a discernible pattern, it is important to assess the person's ability to manage the activities of daily living in his or her own room. A good way to begin this first step in the assessment is to have the person walk around the room. Can he or she walk from a favorite chair to the bathroom with relative ease? Rearranging the furniture may help the person move about the room more safely. For instance, people with Parkinson's disease usually need open space in their rooms, because once they are in motion they have trouble slowing down to change direction so that they can maneuver around furniture. Conversely, people with severe arthritis may need to have all of their furniture placed close together to offer support as they walk.

Bed Height Adjustment

The second step in the assessment is to have the patient or resident get into and out of bed. If the bed is too high to allow the person's feet to touch the ground when he or she is sitting on the side of the bed, the bed's wheels may need to be removed. Fire regulations should be checked before this is done, since they vary in different jurisdictions. In some cases, wheels may be removed if the floors are not carpeted. If the facility is purchasing new beds, it should consider beds that can be positioned even lower than the current standard hospital bed height of 24 inches. Because bed height is a common problem, some long-term care facilities have placed the resident's mattress on the floor or have used a "Hollywood bed," whose mattress is only a few inches off the floor. This alternative may prevent injuries caused by falling from the bed. However, one must also consider the possibility that staff may be injured when giving personal care, when turning the resident in bed, or when transferring the resident from the bed. Another possibility is to place mats or foam mattresses around the bed. This is a safe way to break a fall if a resident who cannot walk falls from the bed. However, this alternative is not safe for ambulatory residents, since they may slip or trip on the mats. If a resident can walk and tends to get out of bed at night, the caregiver should consider lowering the siderails for easy exit. If the resident's gait is unstable, it may be necessary to install an alarm system to alert the nursing staff that the resident is getting up (see the section of this chapter entitled "Alarms").

Use of Siderails

Siderails are not always appropriate for all patients or residents. Patients or residents who can walk and want to get out of bed by themselves should not be required to have their siderails up. When siderails are used, half siderails rather than three-quarter or full siderails should be considered. The patient or resident can use half siderails to pull up to a sitting position. Such rails protect the person from rolling out of bed accidentally without encumbering his or her ability to get out of bed at will. This is helpful to the older adult who needs to get to the bathroom quickly during the night. Half siderails also decrease the person's likelihood of climbing over the siderail and falling, a situation whose injury potential is much higher than merely sliding off the side of the bed. If it is not feasible to purchase half siderails, then it may be best to stop using siderails altogether for some patients or residents. The OBRA guidelines discourage the use of siderails when the patient or resident has no obvious need for them.

Use of Grab-Bars

The third step in the assessment is to evaluate the patient's or resident's ability to get on and off the toilet independently and safely. Grab-bars mounted beside the toilet may be needed for further stability. Some facilities mount their towel racks in concrete, since older people tend to grab them for support (Lewis, 1990).

Use of Nonslip Strips

It is important to note what occurs when the patient or resident gets up from the toilet. Often the person's feet tend to slide when rising. Nonslip strips placed on the floor directly in front of the toilet help the person's feet grip when attempting to stand. These strips are also helpful for older adults who tend to lose bladder continence when trying to sit down on the toilet. The strips prevent slippage when the floor is wet from urine. Placing these strips on the floor beside these residents' beds is also helpful. Scotch Tred℠ by 3M is a nonslip strip that can be used to prevent slipping even when the floor is wet. These strips tend to adhere better to a tile floor than to a ceramic one. Nonslip strips should be laid by the maintenance and/or environmental services department according to the manufacturer's suggestions. To decide how many strips to place, the patient or resident should get up from the bed or toilet and take four to six steps. The strips should be placed approximately every 6 inches for that distance.

Lighting

Because of the aging eye's decreased sensitivity to light, all older patients or residents should have night lights. Night lights not only help them find the bathroom, but also help them orient themselves to their surroundings. Glare becomes a significant problem for older people because of visual changes. Curtains or shades help decrease glare and facilitate vision during daylight hours, thus making the environment safer.

Hallways

Environmental adaptations are limited by the facility's architectural design and by the cost of modifications. Some areas, such as hallways, cannot be altered, but they can be made safer. Equipment and clutter in hallways present real dangers to a frail, older patient or resident who must depend upon the wall rails for support when walking. Staff should be reminded of this periodically.

For many older adults, long hallways tend to appear distorted. This distortion can be reduced by placing chairs in strategic locations. This decreases the tunnel effect of long hallways and gives the person a place to rest when walking.

Shiny floors may look pretty to visitors, but they present a terrible hazard to older people. Because they look wet, such floors may cause concern for patients or residents who are afraid of falling. Moreover, these floors are often slippery. The housekeeping department should be told not to use wax or floor cleaner that promotes a shine, since floors that shine are simply another environmental hazard for the older adults.

Visual Barriers To Prevent Unauthorized Entry by Patients or Residents Who Wander

The fact that some patients or residents with dementia wander is often cited as another reason to use restraints (Evans & Strumpf, 1989). It is helpful if staff members can take a relaxed attitude toward wandering. (Chapter 11 examines some facets of wandering behavior.)

Although staff may become more comfortable with older adults who wander, the more mentally intact patients or residents may not. Some of them may become upset when a "lost" person wanders into their room. A fabric strip, placed across the doorway and covering the doorknob, has been shown to prevent those who wander from entering a room (Namazi, Rosner, & Calkins, 1989). An 18-inch strip of yellow vinyl has also been shown to be an effective visual barrier (McGovern, Duckett, & Learn, 1987). However, a strip this wide is often too cumbersome even for the mentally intact patient or resident to remove when entering his or her own room. A 3-inch strip of fabric, attached to the door's frame with Velcro™ and placed at the same level as the doorknob, has been shown to keep most patients or residents who wander from entering other people's rooms. The narrow strip is easy for the mentally intact person to release and replace at will, whereas the wandering patient or resident usually moves on when confronted with this strip. Both yellow and red strips have been used, and color does not appear to be a significant factor. Doors that lead to kitchens, stairwells, or other areas where only staff may enter or exit may require a wider fabric barrier. Towels may also be hung on exit doors to disguise them so that a patient or resident with dementia will bypass the door rather than attempt to leave through it.

Seating

Seating is another facet of the environment that needs to be considered when removing restraints. Many residents in long-term care facilities spend a large portion of the day sitting in wheelchairs. (See Glickstein, 1988, for a good reference on wheelchairs and sitting posture.) Yet, wheelchairs were not designed for long-term sitting. They were designed for transport only. Residents should be repositioned frequently and alternative seating should be used as much as possible if the person must remain seated. Proper seating is essential for the resident's well-being. A resident who is seated improperly, and therefore uncomfortably, is more likely to try to get out of the chair or wheelchair unassisted, making him or her more likely to be restrained.

Correct wheelchair positioning and proper use of chairs designed for older adults can help ensure safe seating and thus help caregivers avoid the use of restraints. This is particularly important in view of the 1987 OBRA regulations, but it is also imperative from the standpoint of providing care. However, before the caregiver examines the various postural supports that may be used as safe alternatives to wheelchair restraints, he or she must understand correct postural alignment.

Correct postural alignment can only be achieved by proper pelvic positioning. When a person is seated, the pelvis serves as the foundation for the trunk, head, and limbs. In a proper sitting position, the pelvis is in a slight anterior tilt. This position maintains correct alignment of the spine, head, and trunk, and allows weight to be distributed equally over the ischial tuberosities. The legs act as a stable base for the seated person and therefore must be supported properly. The feet should rest on a flat surface and the hips, knees, and ankles each should be flexed at approximately a 90° angle (see Figure 6.1). When the pelvis and feet are positioned thus, the trunk and head will be aligned correctly (Glickstein, 1988).

Stationary Chairs It is important to provide appropriate alternative seating for patients and residents. This means selecting chairs

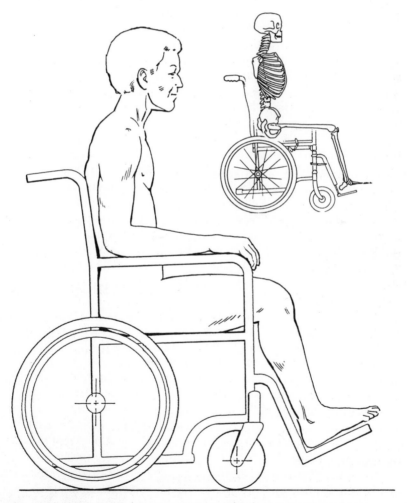

Figure 6.1. Correct postural alignment while seated in wheelchair. The pelvis is tilted slightly backward. The hips, knees, and ankles are flexed at a 90° angle.

with the proper dimensions to support the person when seated and to allow him or her to sit and stand safely. Stationary chairs, rockers, and recliners should be available. Although one chair style will not suit every patient or resident, a few basic dimensions should be evaluated when the caregiver chooses chairs for the facility. The following dimensions may be used as guidelines for chair selection:

Arm height—7 inches above the top of the seat
Seat height—18 inches from the floor to the top of the seat
Seat width—19 inches between the arms
Seat depth—18–19 inches

Wheelchairs   The caregiver should always keep in mind that wheelchairs are a means of transportation and should not be used for sitting. Patients or residents should be seated in appropriate stationary chairs after reaching their destination. However, when a wheelchair is used, it must fit the individual properly or correct postural alignment cannot be maintained (Glickstein, 1988). The seat width, depth, height, and footrests must be evaluated (see Figures 6.2 and 6.3).

Seat Width   The seat width determines whether or not the person will be supported adequately (Glickstein, 1988). The caregiver should be able to slide a hand between the side panel of the armrests and the person's hips (a clearance of about 1 inch). If this is not possible, the chair is too narrow, and the person's skin may break down as a result. If the chair is too wide, the person's trunk will be unstable and he or she may tend to lean or fall to one side (see Figure 6.2).

Seat Depth   The ideal seat depth supports the weight of the trunk and thighs and allows the person to sit upright with a neutral or slightly anterior pelvic tilt (Glickstein, 1988). A seat that is too deep places the pelvis in a posterior tilt position. This will increase pressure on the ischial tuberosities and cause sacral and thoracolumbar skin breakdown. Sitting in a posterior tilt position for an extended period of time may cause decreased range of motion in the hip and lumbar region, increased pressure on buttocks and feet, structural spinal deformities, and impaired arm and leg function. To achieve the anterior pelvic tilt position, there should be a clearance of three or four fingers width (2–3 inches) between the posterior skin crease of the person's knee and the edge of the seat. The seat must be deep enough to provide proper thigh support. A seat that is too deep can force the person's pelvis into a posterior tilt position and cause him or her to slide forward out of the chair (see Figure 6.4).

Seat Height   A seat of the proper height supports the person's feet and thighs adequately and prevents increased pressure on the

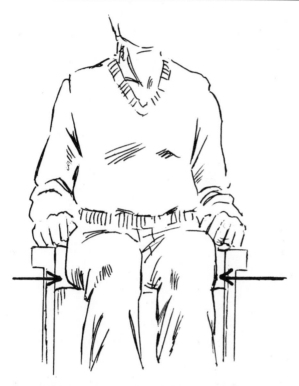

Figure 6.2. Proper width of a wheelchair. The palm of the hand should fit between the person's hip and the side of the chair. This allows a clearance of approximately 1 inch between the hip and the chair. No pressure should be necessary to insert the hand, which should touch the person's hip and the side of the chair.

heels, buttocks, and popliteal areas (see Figure 6.3). The feet should rest flat on the floor or on the footrests. The foot-to-leg angle should be approximately 90°. This also flexes the hips and knees at a 90° angle and allows the thighs to rest parallel to the seat. If the person uses his or her feet to propel the wheelchair, the seat should be at the appropriate height to allow the person to sit with the feet flat on the floor while maintaining proper postural alignment. When the seat is too high, the person will need to move forward in the chair to use his or her feet. This will result in a posterior pelvic tilt and the person will be more likely to fall out of the chair (Glickstein, 1988).

Footrests All patients or residents who do not use their feet to propel the wheelchair should have a wheelchair equipped with footrests. Heel loops may be used to keep the person's feet from sliding off the footrests. Footrests provide the proper support for pelvic alignment, protect the feet from injury, reduce pressure on the

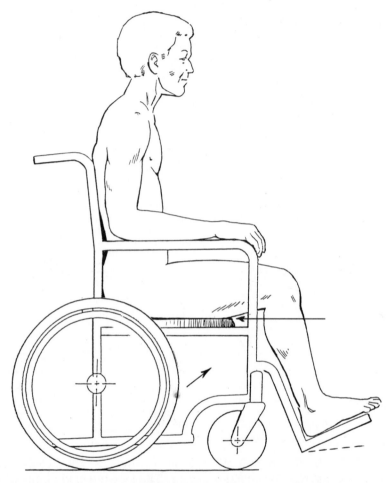

Figure 6.3. Proper seat height of a wheelchair. The lowest part of the footrest should be at least 2 inches from the floor. This provides a clearance at the front of the seat of approximately 1½–2 inches. The caregiver should be able to slip his or her fingers under the person's thigh to a depth of two knuckles at the front of the seat.

thighs, and minimize circulatory complications that may result when the feet are left unsupported. The height of the footrests should be adjusted so that the person's thighs are in a straight line with the supporting surface. There should be at least a 2-inch clearance above the floor in order to prevent the footrest from hitting uneven surfaces. The caregiver should be able to slide his or her fingers gently between the patient's or resident's thigh and the front of the seat cushion for a distance of 1½–2 inches (see Figure 6.3).

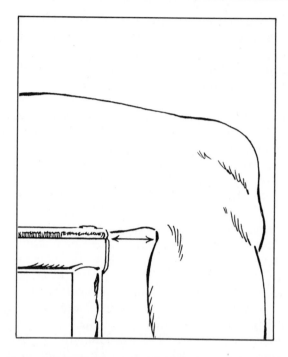

Figure 6.4. Proper seat depth of a stationary chair or wheelchair should be approximately 18 inches. The space between the front edge of the seat upholstery and the area behind the knee should be approximately 2 inches.

Like a seat that is too narrow, footrests that are too high force the person's knees up, placing weight on the ischium, causing skin breakdown. If the footrests are too low, increased pressure against the back of the person's legs will compromise blood flow to the legs (Glickstein, 1988).

Wheelchair Cushions The wheelchair cushion provides the platform for the person to perform daily tasks. Selecting the most appropriate wheelchair cushion is as essential as choosing the proper wheelchair (Glickstein, 1988). The wheelchair cushion improves comfort, promotes stable posture, absorbs shock during propulsion, and prevents skin breakdown. The selection of a seat cushion is not a simple process; no single cushion meets the needs of all clients. The standard sling seat and back of most wheelchairs do not provide adequate support. As the upholstery stretches with time, the person tends to sink into the middle of the chair, causing the pelvis to tilt posteriorly. Sling seats also fail to provide adequate pressure relief for the patient or resident. A solid seat insert that provides adequate support may be made out of plywood at nominal cost (see Figure 6.5a and the section entitled "Construction of Wheelchair Adaptations").

Back Supports and Back Height   A firm back support provides lateral stability, minimizes spinal deformities, and reduces slouching in the wheelchair. For the resident or patient to be able to propel the wheelchair, shoulder girdle motion cannot be restricted. For this reason, the top edge of the seatback must be below the interior angle of the scapula (see Figure 6.6). Proper back support is essential for good trunk control. In order to provide additional back support, a solid back may be used (see Figure 6.5b). However, a solid back may not work for an older person with fixed structural postural deformities, such as a kyphosis. In this case, the caregiver must look for other positioning tools, which are examined later.

Wheelchair Armrests   The chair's armrest should be 1 inch above the elbow with the arm hanging at the client's side while seated in the wheelchair (Figure 6.6). Proper armrest height is necessary to prevent joint dislocations, pain, and contractures. The optimal height is one at which the person's arms are supported without elevating or depressing the scapula. Armrests that are too low cause the person to lean to one side or forward for support. Armrests that are too high force the shoulders up as the client leans on the arms for support. This creates an unnatural position and restricts shoulder range of motion. The person's posture should be as correct as his or her disability allows. A paralyzed arm may be positioned on an arm trough instead of a lap board so that the person retains freedom of movement (Figure 6.7). The arm should be positioned so that the elbow is slightly in front of the shoulder, with the forearm resting perpendicular to the back of the wheelchair and the wrist in neutral position. The hand should be kept open, with the thumb positioned to the side. An increase in muscle tone may cause the hand to tighten, the elbow to flex, and the forearm to move toward the body. Patients or residents and staff alike should be instructed to reposition the person's hand if this occurs (Glickstein, 1988). A half tray can also be used to provide upper extremity support, without restricting the mobility of the resident (Figure 6.8). Fine motor activities can be mounted on the half trays. This may provide diversional activities that can prevent the resident from leaning forward out of the chair.

Common Wheelchair Seating Problems   Often, older patients or residents have musculoskeletal problems that prevent them from sitting upright in a wheelchair, even when positioned properly. This can present the caregiver with the challenge of providing safe,

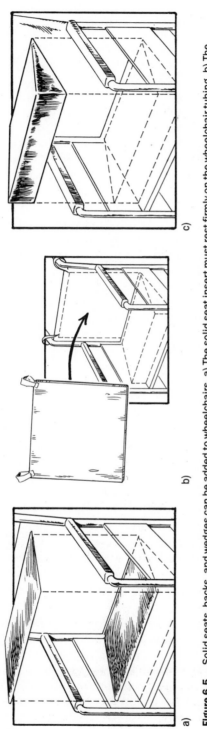

Figure 6.5. Solid seats, backs, and wedges can be added to wheelchairs. a) The solid seat insert must rest firmly on the wheelchair tubing. b) The solid back can be attached to the wheelchair by attaching Naugahyde loops to the corners of the back and hanging them on the wheelchair hand grips. c) A solid wedge seat can be used in place of a solid flat seat for residents who have a tendency to slide out of their chairs.

a)

b)

c)

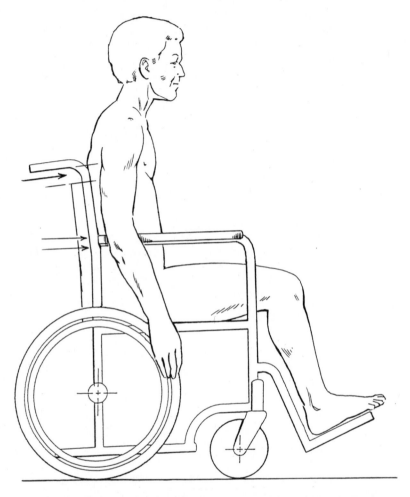

Figure 6.6. The armrest of the wheelchair should be 1 inch higher than the person's elbow when the arm is hanging at the person's side. The caregiver should be able to insert four or five fingers between the patient's armpit and the top of the back upholstery, touching both at the same time.

comfortable seating without the use of restraints. Table 6.1 lists some common seating problems and some restorative care solutions that have been found to be helpful. The next section of this chapter describes how to construct some of these adaptations. The other equipment shown in the table may be purchased from a local durable equipment company.

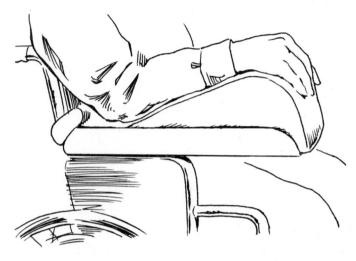

Figure 6.7. An arm trough can be used instead of a lap board for patients or residents with paralyzed arms, thus allowing freedom of movement. The hand is elevated to prevent edema.

Construction of Wheelchair Adaptations

Solid Wheelchair Seat A solid seat insert can prevent the posterior pelvic tilt created by the typical sling seat of a wheelchair. A solid wheelchair seat, shown in Figure 6.5a, can be constructed from half-inch plywood. To do so, cut an 18″ × 16″ rectangle for a standard adult wheelchair, or 16″ × 16″ square for a narrow adult wheelchair. Cover the board with Naugahyde, securing it with staples. Place the finished piece on top of the wheelchair seat tubing. Make certain that the solid seat insert rests firmly on the wheelchair tubing or it will not give adequate support and will tip when the person gets out of the chair. Place a cushion appropriate for the person's condition on top of the plywood for comfort and pressure relief.

Solid Back A firm back, shown in Figure 6.5b, provides stability and helps keep the person in an upright posture in the wheelchair. To make a solid back, follow the procedure for constructing a solid seat. Place Naugahyde loops on two corners of the back piece to secure it to the wheelchair's handgrips. When positioning patients or residents with fixed structural deformities, a solid back may not be appropriate. Often, a foam piece cut to conform to the person's deformities is needed instead of or in addition to the solid back to give adequate support.

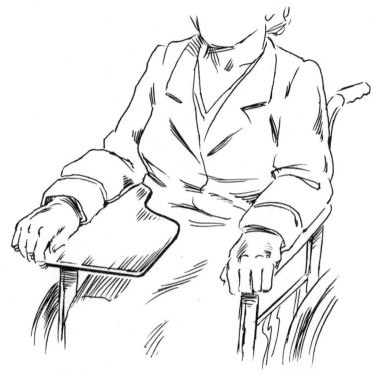

Figure 6.8. A half tray can be used to support the upper extremity while allowing freedom of movement.

Half-Moon Footrest Extension Often, a patient or resident may have difficulty keeping his or her feet on the footrests. When this happens, the person loses support for the lower extremities and may slide out of the wheelchair. Even if the person does not slide out, he or she may still suffer breakdown in the skin of the lower thighs and/or buttocks. In the past, toe loops were used to help solve this problem. The use of the half-moon extension provides an extended support surface that allows the person's feet to remain on the wheelchair without the use of toe loop restraints. To construct the half-moon extension, cut a semicircle of half-inch plywood with a 14-inch base and a 13-inch height (see Figure 6.9). Cover it with nonslip material or Naugahyde and place a nonslip strip across the top surface. Secure the half-moon to one of the wheelchair's footrests with a screw. This allows the footrests to be removed or swung away for safe transfers.

Lateral Supports Lateral supports allow the person who has poor control of the trunk muscles to remain upright in the wheel-

Table 6.1. Common wheelchair seating problems

Problem	Solution
Person leans forward	Reclined wheelchair position. Often, a recline of 15°–30° will eliminate the need for a chest restraint to prevent forward trunk slouching. Reclining removes the effects of gravity and minimizes the amount of muscle control and strength needed to maintain an upright posture.
Person leans to the side	Lateral support (see Figure 6.9)
Feet slip off footrests	Half-moon foot extension (see Figure 6.9)
Legs fall backward off footrests or between calf pads	Leg panel (see Figure 6.11)
Arm falls over side of wheelchair/ shoulder becomes subluxed	Arm trough or half-tray (see Figures 6.7 and 6.8)
Head falls forward or backward	Head extension/reclined wheelchair position (see Figure 6.10)
Person slides out of wheelchair	Wedge seat (see Figure 6.5c)
Wheelchair tilts forward or backward	Antitippers
Person reaches forward to play with clothes or shoes	Half-tray with activity

chair without the use of a chest restraint. To construct such a support, cut out a square or rectangular piece of ½-inch plywood. The specific needs and postural problems of the patient or resident will determine the size of the support. Pad the board and cover it with Naugahyde, securing it to the sides of the wheelchair back with metal brackets. Place the brackets in a position that allows the person some lateral mobility but that is close enough to the person's body to prevent him or her from being injured by falling to the side (see Figure 6.9).

Wedge Seat The solid wedge seat can decrease the person's risk of sliding out of the chair. However, it may increase the risk of pressure ulcers on the sacral area. If a wedge seat is used, this risk needs to be addressed. To make the insert shown in Figure 6.5c, cut a 2-inch piece of plywood into 3- by 3-inch squares. Attach these wooden blocks to the two front corners of the solid seat insert. Make sure the blocks rest on the wheelchair seat tubing. The height of the blocks can be varied to provide greater pelvic tilt, decreasing the person's risk of sliding out of the chair.

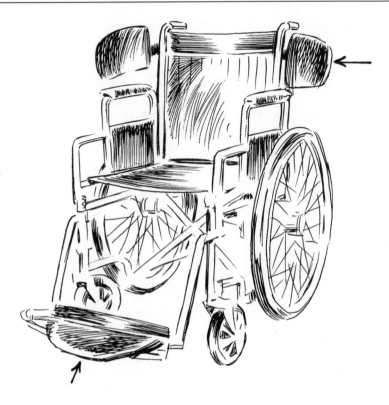

Figure 6.9. A half-moon extension to a wheelchair provides an extended support surface that allows the feet to remain on the wheelchair pedal without the need for toe loop restraints. Lateral supports can be used to provide additional trunk support.

ACTIVITIES AS AN ALTERNATIVE TO RESTRAINTS

Activities play a major role in creating a restorative care environment. Involvement in purposeful activity relieves boredom and thus can diminish the restlessness that often leads older patients and residents to wander aimlessly and to attempt to get up unassisted. Activities should meet both physiological and psychosocial needs. Therapeutic physical exercise can help improve and maintain muscle strength so that the person can continue to walk and to perform the activities of daily living. Cognitive stimulation not only improves mental outlook but can distract the person from pursuing nonpurposeful and unsafe behaviors.

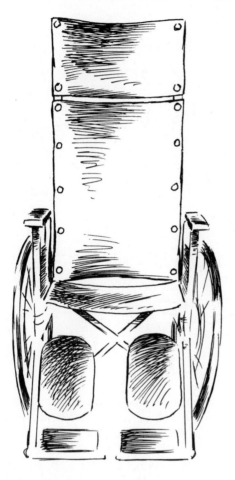

Figure 6.10. A head extension can be added to the wheelchair to prevent the head from leaning backward.

Whether physical or mental, therapeutic activities that focus on the person's interests and his or her care needs are most effective in reducing the use of restraints. An exchange of information among all departments is essential to the care planning process. Such an exchange allows the activities department to create care plans that complement those of other departments.

An example of how the activities department can help develop alternatives to restraint use involves the resident who frequently tries to get out of the wheelchair without help. If the suggested

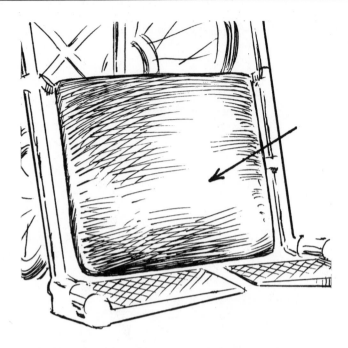

Figure 6.11. A leg panel can be used to prevent the legs from falling backward off the footrests or between the calf pads.

wheelchair adaptations have been added but have not prevented the person from trying to get up, the activities department might try to develop a program of therapeutic exercise and cognitive stimulation. Therapeutic group exercise expands the efforts of physical therapy and nursing to increase leg strength. Eventually, this may help the person become able to walk independently. Group exercise also offers the person another structured opportunity to get out of the wheelchair. Cognitive stimulation may take the form of diversionary activities. The person whose interest is absorbed in a craft project may be satisfied to remain in a chair when staff members are unavailable to help him or her walk.

One function of nursing is to communicate the resident's needs to the activities staff and help them find the appropriate activities. A second function is to help the activities department carry out the plan by having the person ready to attend group activities. Nursing staff may also supplement the activities department's role by providing activities on the unit when the activities staff is unavailable. For instance, unit activities, such as a ball toss or crafts, require few nursing staff and are very helpful to patients or residents who tend to become restless when they have no specific activity to attend.

Chapter 12 presents more information on the role of activities in a restorative care setting.

Another strategy that may be helpful in the care planning process is to compile a list of therapeutic groups offered by various departments throughout the facility. Such a list can help the care team identify as many appropriate activities as possible for residents, and it also increases the team's awareness of other departments' offerings in the way of resident activities.

RESPONDING TO PHYSIOLOGICAL CHANGES

Any change in the physiological status of the older person's body has the potential to cause a change in behavior that may lead to restraint use. Some physiological changes that may increase the likelihood of being restrained are shown in Table 6.2. Therefore, addressing or treating the underlying physiological problem becomes a restraint alternative in and of itself. Frequently, older people do not present with the usual symptoms of illness. Often, the first symptoms of a disease process, pain, or an adverse drug reaction is confusion or agitation, incontinence, falling, or immobility (Fox, 1985). It is not uncommon for older people to experience a series of falls rather than a temperature elevation as the presenting symptom of an infectious disease. When an older person's ability to walk suddenly deteriorates, or when he or she has a sudden series of falls, it is imperative that the staff look for the reason that underlies this change rather than apply a restraint which will only treat the symptom. An example of such a situation involves a patient or resident who has been independent in ambulation and who suddenly has a series of unrelated falls over a 3-day period. On the 4th day the resident wakes up with a temperature of 101°F and symptoms of pneumonia. The falls could have been related to the infection. In the past, to prevent injury, the staff may have placed the resident in a restraint; and the underlying cause of the falls might have been overlooked. However, in the restorative care environment, the goal is to question the cause of the falls and attempt to avoid restraint use.

It is beyond the scope of this book to present the spectrum of the older adult's response to physiological changes. The effects of immobility, examined in Chapters 5 and 11, should help the reader to understand the older person's response to illness.

NURSING ALTERNATIVES TO RESTRAINTS

When faced with the prospect of removing restraints, staff members often express concern that the facility has too few nurses to monitor

Table 6.2.   Physiological changes that can lead to restraint use

Change	Explanation/intervention
Agitation and confusion associated with pain	Pain often causes older adults to become agitated and confused. As a consequence, they may attempt to get out of bed, rise from the chair, or wander. The resident or patient should be treated with nonnarcotic analgesics or low-dose narcotic analgesics for short periods of time as needed. Ongoing assessment is required to monitor the presence of pain and the individual's response to the pain medication.
Agitation or restlessness resulting from constipation or incontinence	Older adults who are unable to express their need to use the toilet may become agitated when they experience discomfort from constipation or incontinence. Elimination needs should be monitored by staff and suspected as the cause if there is sudden restlessness for no apparent reason.
Dizziness, loss of balance, or dehydration	Dehydration can lead to low blood pressure upon standing, causing loss of balance and dizziness, and mental confusion in many older people. Dehydration should be suspected in an older person who is taking diuretics, is vomiting or suffering from diarrhea, or is experiencing dizziness, loss of balance, or new onset confusion.
Weakness following an illness	After any acute illness or hospitalization that results in a decrease or loss of functional ability, the patient or resident should be referred for a physical therapy/occupational therapy evaluation.
Disorientation and/or sensory deprivation	Sensory deprivation can be extremely disorienting to a person of any age. Sensory deprivation can occur when sight or hearing is impaired or when mobility is restricted. Staff should make sure

(continued)

Table 6.2. *continued*

Change	Explanation/intervention
	that older patients or residents have easy access to any prescribed aids (glasses, hearing aids, etc.) and that they are wearing them. This fosters a safe, supportive environment and makes the person less likely to need restraints. To increase sensory stimulation, residents should be brought out to the nurses' station. Where possible, intravenous lines should be replaced with heparin locks. Catheters and feeding tubes should be removed as soon as possible. These steps will negate the need to tie the person's hands.
Change in behavior related to medications	Any drug, even a drug that has been used for a long time, has the potential to cause behavioral changes. If there is a change in behavior, all the drugs that a patient or resident is taking should be assessed and monitored for adverse reactions.

safety effectively. Yet, many facilities have decreased the use of restraints without having to increase the staff-to-patient ratios. A restraint-free environment requires that staff time be used differently, not that more staff be used. Many of the alternatives to restraints make use of common nursing interventions, but with an emphasis on observation and anticipation of the patients' or residents' needs.

Toilet Schedules

Nurses often strive to toilet patients or residents on a regular schedule; in the restraint-free environment, toileting schedules take on particular importance. Regular toileting meets the older adult's physiological need for elimination and thus may lessen his or her restlessness or agitation. At the same time, a toileting schedule allows the nursing staff some control over the times at which a patient or resident is likely to try to get up unassisted. This intervention is helpful even when the person is incontinent, because a patient or resident who regularly is kept dry and comfortable is less likely to get up unassisted.

Although 2-hour toilet intervals tend to be the norm, other schedules can work equally well. Many nursing assistants have found that giving the patient or resident a chance to use the toilet before and/or after meals and at bedtime is sufficient. Older people who try to get out of bed at night should be assisted to use the toilet at 11:00 P.M. and again at 4:00 A.M. Many falls occur between 12:00 A.M. and 2:00 A.M. and again between the hours of 5:00 A.M. and 7:00 A.M. Assisting a patient or resident to use the toilet before high-risk times anticipates the need for elimination and also meets the need for adequate sleep. Helping the person walk to the toilet rather than use a bedpan allows him or her to empty the bladder completely, thereby increasing the likelihood of success with this intervention.

Daily Physical Ambulation

For older adults who are physically able to walk, regular ambulation can improve their gait and weight-bearing ability. In turn, those who walk at regular intervals may, in time, become independent in ambulation and may no longer need to be restrained. In others, for whom walking independently is an unlikely goal, frequent assisted walking can strengthen muscles so that the person will not fall immediately upon standing up. These few seconds of independent standing can give staff time to reach the person and provide whatever assistance he or she needs. Walking at regular intervals throughout the day also meets the person's need for activity and relieves boredom. A person who exercises regularly is less restless and less likely to try to get up without help.

One way to ensure that patients' and residents' need for regular exercise is met is to develop a nurse-administered walking program that is based on daily goals. A rehabilitation nurse or charge nurse can assess the gait of each patient or resident who is capable of walking but is not safe to do so alone, and set an appropriate goal. In facilities where there is no rehabilitation nurse, the physical therapy department can be consulted. Making the walking goal part of the care plan and holding the primary nursing assistant accountable for documenting that the patient or resident was assisted to walk can help promote regular ambulation for those who are frail.

Observation

Observation does not require more nursing staff, but it does require that the existing staff members understand that this intervention is necessary to help keep patients or residents from falling. Staff members may see patients or residents frequently during the day without truly observing them. Frequent accurate observation requires that staff members must think about what they are seeing and anticipate the patient's or resident's needs. If observation is called for, staff members are more likely to comply if they understand that the purpose of this intervention is to help keep the patient or resident from falling.

Keeping patients or residents out of their rooms and within sight of the nurses' station is one way of observing them. Patients and residents who are left alone in their rooms are likely to fall if they attempt to meet their own needs. When a patient or resident is in a more public area, staff members have an opportunity to notice if the person is getting restless or needs something. Observation may also mean checking on patients or residents every hour, both at night and during the day, to make sure that those whose behavior is unpredictable do not get up without help. Residents or patients who tend to fall when using the toilet or performing self-care tasks may need frequent observation in the course of these activities to ensure their safety.

Tracking

Tracking is similar to observation but it is an intervention that is designed specifically for patients or residents who wander. In this intervention, the staff member notes the patient's or resident's location hourly. An hourly tracking sheet, with space for a check mark or the staff member's initials, is placed on the patient's or resident's door to encourage staff members to be aware of the person's location.

Alarms

There are times when observation and tracking are insufficient for monitoring patients or residents. In such cases, many facilities have used alarms successfully. Using an alarm can reassure the staff that they have a tool to help them monitor an unpredictable person when restraints are no longer an option. Families may also feel reassured when an alarm is used temporarily on a patient or resident who previously had been restrained. Facilities that have used alarms have reported a decrease in the number of falls (Chenitz, Kussman, & Stone, 1991; Kleyman, 1992; Widder, 1985). Alarms are most successful when used to monitor patients or residents who are strong enough to get up without help but who are likely to fall because their gait is unstable or because they lack the memory and/or judgment to summon help when they need it. Often, those who benefit from the use of alarms are people who were previously ambulating independently but who, because of an acute illness, are no longer able to do so. The alarm signal not only summons the nursing staff but also reminds the patient or resident to wait for help.

Alarms should not be used on agitated patients or residents, because their body movements will cause frequent "false alarms" that may discourage the nursing staff from answering the alarm right away. Successful alarm use requires that staff limit alarm use to patients or residents for whom it will truly be beneficial, and that they have the person's cooperation. If the care team is considering an alarm, the patient or resident must be consulted first, since some older people may dislike the idea of being "attached" to an alarm.

Many types of alarms are now available, and a facility that is considering using an alarm system should research them thoroughly. A facility may choose to use more than one type of alarm to meet different patients' or residents' needs. Caregivers should exercise caution not to use too many alarms or to become too dependent on them. If there are too many alarms in use on one unit, staff members may become less aware of their sound. It is important to remind staff members that alarms do not replace alert observation, but are meant to be used as a tool to help keep patients and residents safe.

Napping

Whenever an older adult is restrained because he or she falls out of a chair while asleep, napping in bed is an appropriate restraint alternative. Napping is important to anyone who is chairbound. The change in position from chair to bed is necessary to ensure the person's comfort as well as health. The key is to observe when the person will benefit most from this rest. Some people are slow to get going in the morning and may need a nap after breakfast. Others may need a nap after lunch or later in the afternoon. Still others need rest breaks in both the morning and the afternoon. Nursing assistants usually know what time of day a patient or resident reaches his or her low point, but they may feel uncomfortable letting the person nap if it is not a part of the unit's usual routine. An individualized care plan, which is central to a restorative care environment, allows these specific needs to be met.

Drug Evaluation

Chapter 10 of this book examines in detail the effects of psychotropic drugs used as chemical restraints on older adults. However, all drugs potentially can affect older people adversely and therefore may be implicated in causing behavior that may lead to restraint use. A number of drugs that produce few or no side effects in younger people may cause changes in an older adult's mental status. These side effects can mean the difference between the person's being restrained for safety and his or her remaining safely unrestrained. Therefore, when a caregiver is considering either removing or using a restraint, it is imperative to consider the possible negative effects of all medications.

Resident Education

Many residents of long-term care facilities lack short-term memory and/or judgment. Nevertheless, many of them respond well to frequent reminders not to get up without help. Throughout the shift, the nursing assistant can remind these residents to call for help if they need to get up. The nursing staff can give unrestrained residents almost hourly reminders as the staff members go about their daily routines and pass residents in the hall. For many residents whose memories are impaired, such frequent verbal reminders can allow them to remain safely restraint free.

Nursing Assistants' Support

The process of removing patients' or residents' restraints is a difficult one for all involved. The nursing assistants who provide direct care, may feel responsible for the safety of the patients or residents on their unit when restraints are removed. They may also fear that if a patient or resident falls or wanders, they will be held responsible. Members of the nursing assistant staff need constant support to help them meet the needs of unrestrained residents. They also need reassurance that if a patient or resident does fall, they will not be held responsible but rather will be asked to contribute their expertise to finding other alternatives to restraints.

CONCLUSION

Since the passage of OBRA '87, numerous products have been developed and marketed as alternatives to restraints. However, many of these products do not provide individualized interventions that enhance the older person's functional ability and independence. Restraints can be removed safely by finding the appropriate alternative that is individualized to the needs of the patient or resident. By modifying the environment, using activities, treating underlying physiological factors and seeking nursing care alternatives, the clinician can develop a care plan that addresses the behavior for which a restraint was used. Creating an environment that promotes physiological and psychosocial well-being is the goal in finding the appropriate restraint alternative.

REFERENCES

Chenitz, W., Kussman, H., & Stone, J. (1991). Preventing falls. In W. Chenitz, J. Stone, & S. Salisbury (Eds.), *Clinical gerontological nursing: A guide to advance practice* (pp. 309–323). Philadelphia: W.B. Saunders.

Evans, L., & Strumpf, N. (1989). Tying down the elderly: A review of the literature on physical restraint. *Journal of the American Geriatrics Society, 37*, 65–74.

Evans, L., & Strumpf, N. (1990). Myths about elder restraint. *Image: Journal of Nursing Scholarship, 22*(2), 124–128.

Fox, R. (1985). Immunology of aging. In J. Brocklehurst (Ed.), *Textbook of geriatric medicine and gerontology* (2nd ed.) (pp. 92–95). New York: Churchill Livingstone.

Glickstein, K. (1988). Wheelchair positioning of neurologically impaired adults: Avoiding complications. *Focus on geriatric care and rehabilitation* (Vol. 2). Rockville, MD: Aspen Systems.

Kleyman, P. (1992, December–January). Preventing falls–High tech is not enough. *Aging Today*, 15.

Lewis, L. (1990). Toward restraint free nursing homes. *Long Term Currents, 13*(1), 1–7.

McGovern, R., Duckett, D., & Learn, L. (1987). What do nursing homes do with wanderers? *AAHA Provider News, 2*(20), 9.

Namazi, K., Rosner, T., & Calkins, M. (1989). Visual barriers to prevent ambulating Alzheimer's patients from exiting through an emergency door. *The Gerontologist, 29*(5), 699–702.

Widder, B. (1985, September/October). A new device to decrease falls. *Geriatric Nursing*, 287–288.

Chapter 7

Nursing Care of the Resident Who Is Physically Restrained

Mary Macholl Kaufmann and May L. Wykle

The practice of using physical restraints is currently under intense scrutiny. No longer can physical restraints be considered a routine, permanent, appropriate, or unquestioned intervention for older adults in long-term care settings. Public outrage over the indiscriminate use of physical restraints began in the 1980s as mounting evidence indicated that the use of these devices was not benign. Serious physical, emotional, and social or behavioral consequences have resulted from the inappropriate use of restraints, especially with older adults. These consequences are considerable, and they reinforce both the need for change in existing restraint practices and the importance of consistent nursing care when restraints are the only alternative. Hence, the opportunity now exists to establish new criteria for the use of physical restraints for frail older adults and to develop new comprehensive care plans.

This chapter examines the appropriate and humane care that older adults in long-term care facilities require when other measures fail and the caregiver must use restraints. The first section examines a person-centered care philosophy as the foundation upon which a restorative care environment rests. The second section provides guidelines for using physical restraints in long-term care facilities. The third section examines nursing care requirements for residents who require brief periods of physical restraint. The last two sections suggest intervention and evaluation techniques.

PERSON-CENTERED PHILOSOPHY OF CARE

The long-term care facility is both a home and a treatment center for older adults that is closely regulated by state and federal authorities. The challenge for the interdisciplinary team in a long-term care setting is to create a home-like environment within which frail and disabled older adults may receive high-quality care and experience optimal quality of life. The goals of long-term care are based on the resident's individualized needs. They include the establishment of a physical environment that is clean and comfortable and that fosters the resident's successful adjustment and independence, as well as the establishment of a psychosocial environment that supports the resident's dignity, right to self-determination, sense of well-being, and feelings of self-worth (Kaufmann, in press).

Evans, Strumpf, and Williams (1991) refer to such individualized care as "person-centered care." Person-centered care is based on the uniqueness of each resident's physical, emotional, psychosocial, cultural, and spiritual needs. Evans and colleagues also believe that the interdisciplinary care team must incorporate each of the

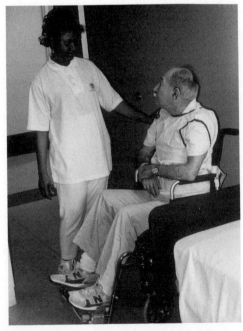

During the time that a physical restraint is used, staff must observe and assess residents or patients frequently to ensure their physical and psychosocial well-being. (Photograph courtesy of the Hebrew Home of Greater Washington. Used by permission.)

values in the list that follows into their care philosophy in order to make the ideal of person-centered care a reality:

1. Opportunities for choice in care decisions
2. Independence, and the strengthening of independence, in every aspect of daily living
3. The right of residents to take risks
4. The importance of relationships and their continuity for residents and staff
5. The practice of an interdisciplinary team approach with an integral role for the nursing assistant
6. Home-like qualities and relative quiet in the physical environment
7. Creativity by staff and residents in problem solving
8. Education of, and partnership with, families (Evans et al. 1991, p. 95)

Hence, the commonplace use of physical restraints becomes incompatible with the goals of individualized, person-centered care. Ideally, physical restraints rarely will need to be used in facilities that emphasize individualized care. Accurate assessment of the resident's needs, continuous monitoring of his or her health and functional status, appropriate adjustments in the resident's care plan, and implementation of innovative alternatives to restraints are actions that caregivers may take to promote a restorative care environment (Stilwell, 1988; Strumpf & Evans, 1991).

GUIDELINES FOR USING PHYSICAL RESTRAINTS

Guidelines for the use of physical restraints generally are based on either the facility's mission statement or the nursing department's philosophy statement. Mission or philosophy statements are written documents that clearly delineate for an interdisciplinary team the facility's principles of care and that serve as the foundation for the facility's policies and procedures. Appendix 7.A of this chapter provides a sample philosophy of care statement for the nursing department of a long-term care facility.

The facility's policies and procedures reflect not only the principles of care outlined in the mission or philosophy statements, but also current standards of practice. The American Nurses Association (ANA) publishes standards of practice for nurses that define the responsibilities for which the profession believes its practitioners are accountable. The ANA's standards of practice that apply specifically to nurses who work with older adults are found in the *Standards and Scope of Gerontological Nursing Practice* (1987). The standards it presents are intended to be used in conjunction with other ANA documents, such as *Standards of Rehabilitation Nursing,* the *Code of Conduct,* and the recently revised *Standards of Clinical Nursing Practice.* Together, these standards provide guidance for nurses who practice in long-term care facilities and also help shape decisions related to the use of physical restraints. In addition, the Omnibus Budget Reconciliation Act (OBRA) of 1987 outlines a set of federal standards pertaining to the use of physical restraints.

Evans et al. (1991) have summarized seven standards of care for restraint use from an extensive review of the literature. In general, physical restraints should:

1. be used only on a short-term basis and as a last resort [after other less restrictive interventions have failed];
2. [be applied] by staff properly trained in their use;
3. trigger further investigation and treatment aimed at elimination of the problem causing the need for restraint; . . .
4. be applied only as a result of collaborative decision-making between nurse, physician, and other health team members; . . .
5. incorporate informed decision-making by patients and families; . . .
6. never [be] used as a substitute for monitoring and surveillance; and
7. require attention to patient comfort and safety during periods of their use. (p. 95)

In addition, the Gerontological Nursing Practice Group of the Massachusetts Nurses Association has developed a set of guidelines for the use of restraints in nonpsychiatric settings to assist nurses in decision making and care planning for residents who need physical restraints (Fulmer, Dix, Yoder, & Terrill, 1983). These guidelines outline the importance of: 1) continual assessment of the resident's physical and psychosocial needs that result from the restraint; 2) the continuous evaluation of expected outcomes of care; and 3) thorough documentation that includes frequent monitoring and assessment, restorative interventions that maintain the resident's highest practical level of physical and psychosocial function, and evaluation of the effectiveness of the physical restraints in achieving the desired outcomes of care for the resident. Appendix 7.B provides an example of a long-term care facility's policy on the use of physical restraints.

NURSING CARE OF THE RESIDENT
WHO IS PHYSICALLY RESTRAINED

In a restorative care environment, the interdisciplinary team must always consider the decision to apply physical restraints as an extraordinary and temporary measure. Restraints should be used only as a last resort when less restrictive approaches have failed. This section examines the nursing care requirements for residents who need temporary physical restraints.

Data Collection

According to the ANA standards (1987), caregivers should perform comprehensive, accurate, systematic health assessments of all residents in the facility. The members of the interdisciplinary care team, the resident, and the resident's family all should have access to the data collected during the assessment.

Ideally, the decision to use physical restraints should be made by the care team whenever possible, because of the many adverse effects associated with the use of physical restraints. Kaufmann (1991) believes that the success of maintaining a restorative care environment depends on a team's creative problem-solving abilities and collaborative efforts. Physical restraints should be considered only after the team has reviewed the health assessment data. To avoid subjective decision-making, the team might make use of a flow chart such as the one developed by Morrison, Crinklaw-Wiancko, King, Thibeault, and Wells (1987) to guide their use of physical restraints (see Figure 7.1). If the team concludes that all other interventions have failed to correct or resolve the resident's problem, they may then decide to use physical restraints. They should also document the failure of previous approaches in the resident's record (American Health Care Association, 1990).

When used temporarily and appropriately, restraints may serve the resident's needs rather than the team's need to maintain control or to punish (American Health Care Association, 1990; Wolanin & Phillips, 1981). Using a physical restraint may be appropriate under the following circumstances:

1. The resident behaves disruptively or violently.
2. The resident reveals the potential for injuring him- or herself or others.
3. The resident is unable to maintain proper body alignment.
4. The resident interferes with his or her medical treatment (Brower, 1991).

Morrison and colleagues (1987) believe that ongoing use of physical restraints requires the team's involvement and agreement. Occasionally, such as on weekends or in emergencies, the nursing staff may have to make the decision to use physical restraints without the benefit of the team's collaboration to solve the problem creatively. In

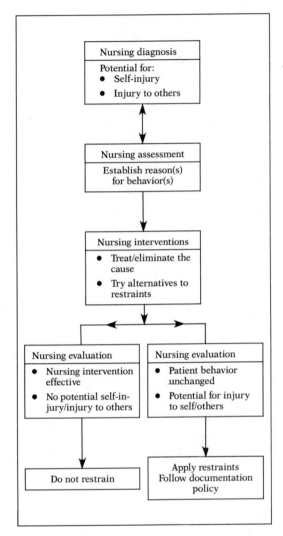

Figure 7.1. Flow chart for deciding whether or not to restrain a resident. (From Morrison, J., Crinklaw-Wiancko, D., King, D., Thibeault, S., & Wells, D.L. [1987]. Formulating a restraint use policy. *Journal of Nursing Administration, 17*[3], 39–42; reprinted by permission.)

these instances, Darby (1990) recommends that the nurse consult with another nurse who is more experienced or knowledgeable, such as a clinical nurse specialist, nurse manager, or nursing supervisor. Requiring that more than one individual be involved in the decision to restrain a resident helps ensure that the facility adheres to its restorative care policy.

Nursing Diagnosis

The nursing diagnosis, which uses data taken from the resident's health assessment, is one of several methods that may be used to categorize residents' problems (American Nurses Association, 1987). The North American Nursing Diagnostic Association (NANDA) developed a system of diagnostic categories, or nursing diagnoses, by which nurses or interdisciplinary teams can formulate a care plan and implement selected interventions based on a thorough assessment of the resident's needs (Gordon, 1987). A nursing diagnosis is a clearly defined statement describing a resident's problem that requires the health care team's intervention. When the team's assessment identifies that the resident's behavior jeopardizes his or her own safety and security needs or that of other residents, a diagnostic category may be identified.

Using the nursing diagnosis technique, the team might describe a problem that requires restraint use in one of the following ways:

1. Potential for injury; several recent falls
2. Intermittent episodes of violence; abuses self and others
3. Altered thought processes; confusion related to drug effects

The team would then document that diagnosis in the resident's care plan.

Planning and Continuity of Care

Goals Two principles are important for the interdisciplinary team to consider when writing the goal or goals of care for residents who are physically restrained. Providing the right balance of comfort, freedom of movement, safety, and independence for the resident during the period of restraint is the major principle that the team must consider (Matteson & McConnell, 1988; Rader & Donius, 1991). This is accomplished by using the least restrictive restraint for a temporary, designated period of time (Rader & Donius, 1991). When the facility's policy does not provide a clear definition of the criteria for selection, the team or a nurse must select the type of physical restraint. Usually, the nurse is familiar with the various types of physical restraints that are available and knows the resident's behavior and needs.

The second principle is to use physical restraints that will not themselves cause the resident to suffer further illness (Rose, 1987). A facility's inservice and staff development program can educate all staff about the numerous adverse side effects that a resident may suffer as a result of physical restraints. The team must devise goals and interventions to prevent these side effects.

The team should also document the goal or desired outcome of physical restraint use. Gordon (1987) defines the term *goal* or *outcome* as "measurable behavior indicating problem resolution or progress toward resolution" (p. 22). For example, the team might document two goals of care for a resident who behaves violently from time to time as follows: 1) the resident will not hurt self or others during an episode of violence, and 2) the resident will have fewer episodes of violence.

Involvement of Resident and Family Occasionally, the resident, a family member, or a legal representative will request that a physical restraint be applied. On other occasions, the team will recommend the restraint. In either case, the resident, family member, or legal representative must be fully informed of the reason for using the restraint, the benefits and drawbacks of the specific type of restraint, and the care the resident will receive during the specified period of restraint. Consent from the resident, family member, or legal representative for the use of physical restraints must also be obtained (American Health Care Association, 1990; Calfee, 1988). The facility may elect to have any of these people sign a written document giving the facility consent to restrain the resident. If the facility does not provide a written document to sign, the appropriate member of the team must instead include a summary of the discussion with the resident, family member, or legal representative and his or her verbal consent in the resident's record (American Health Care Association, 1990).

INTERVENTION

After the team determines the goals of care, it must develop specific interventions to ensure that the resident receives high-quality care. For example, the social services staff may provide counseling as an intervention to give the resident, family member, or legal representative an opportunity to discuss his or her thoughts and feelings about the use of physical restraints. In addition, the therapeutic recreation staff may plan additional one-to-one activities for the resident while he or she is restrained.

When a restraint is used, a written statement indicating all of the following parameters should be drafted:

1. The conditions under which the restraint may be applied
2. The specific type and size of restraint to be applied

3. The frequency with which the resident is to be monitored
4. The frequency with which the resident is to be released from the restraint
5. The type of exercise the resident is to perform during the periods in which the restraint is removed
6. The maximum amount of time the restraint may be used
7. The projected date by which the restraint is to be discontinued

Care During Initial Application of Restraint

Safety of the Resident Physical restraints are used primarily as a safety measure to protect a resident (Calfee, 1988). However, when used improperly, physical restraints can produce serious consequences and may cause permanent injury or even death (Evans et al., 1991; Rose, 1987; Tadsen & Brandt, 1973). Therefore, to ensure residents' safety, it is essential that all facilities have guidelines for using restraints. The U.S. Food and Drug Administration has developed 10 recommendations for the safe use of physical restraint devices (U.S. Food and Drug Administration, 1991). These recommendations are shown in Table 7.1. An 11th recommendation is that physical restraints be applied only by staff who are trained in their use (Evans & Strumpf, 1989).

Regular staff training programs with periodic evaluation are recommended for both licensed nurses and nursing assistants to keep them abreast of the latest developments in restraint reduction and restorative care and to ensure that they have the proper nursing care skills when physical restraints are needed (Calfee, 1988; Katz, Weber, & Dodge, 1981). Companies that manufacture physical restraints usually employ representatives who will present inservice training sessions for staff members who use their products. One company (J.T. Posey Company, Arcadia, CA) even offers group workshops in restraint reduction, alternatives to restraint, and proper use of restraints required by OBRA.

Facilities may also purchase educational materials, such as books and videotapes, as resources for staff training. One such reference book is the *Textbook for Nursing Assistants* by Sorrentino (1992). The chapter entitled "Safety in the Home and Health Care Facility," contains a section on physical restraints that presents important information for staff, including a list of safety measures to follow when caring for a restrained resident, illustrated step-by-step procedures for applying specific types of physical restraints, and an illustration for making a square knot (since, according to Sorrentino, a square knot is the best type of knot to use when securing a restraint because

Table 7.1.   Recommendations for safe use of physical restraints

- Follow good nursing and basic patient care practices.
- Monitor patients and residents frequently, and remove restraints often.
- Apply and adjust devices properly to maintain body alignment and comfort.
- Allow the use of restraints only by prescription and for a strictly defined period.
- Define and communicate a clear facility policy on the use of restraints, covering such issues as appropriate conditions for use and length of time to use restraints.
- Display user instructions in a highly visible location and in foreign languages as necessary.
- Keep accurate patient and resident records on the use of the device, including the reason for use, the type selected, and the length of time it should be used.
- Follow local and state laws regarding these devices.
- Explain why the restraint is necessary to facilitate patients' or residents' and their families' understanding and cooperation.
- Follow the manufacturer's directions for use, including:
  — Selecting the appropriate restraint for the patient's or resident's condition
  — Using the correct size
  — Noting front and back of the device and applying it correctly
  — Tying knots with easily released hitches
  — Securing bed restraints to the bed springs or frame, not to the mattress or bedrails. If the bed is adjustable, secure the restraints to the parts of the bed that move with the person to avoid constricting him or her.

Adapted from U.S. Food and Drug Administration (1991).

it is easy to release in an emergency). Books such as this are excellent reference materials to keep on hand for staff on the nursing unit. When such resources are readily available, all staff members can update their knowledge and skills on restraints.

When possible the nurse should explain the purpose of the physical restraint to the resident, family, and/or legal representative before it is applied (American Health Care Association, 1990). This also gives the staff another opportunity to review the benefits and drawbacks of restraints as well as the kind of care the resident will need to receive while in restraints. However, if a resident's behavior is disruptive and a restraint must be applied quickly, the explanation may follow the application of the restraint. Once the restraint has been applied, the nurse and nursing assistant together assess the resident's comfort and safety needs to ensure that:

1. The proper type and size of restraint has been used.
2. Basic nursing care practices have been implemented, if needed.
3. Appropriate, easily released knots have been tied and secured at the appropriate locations.
4. The nurse call button is within the resident's reach.
5. The resident's body is aligned properly.
6. The restraint secures the resident comfortably.

This assessment period also gives the nurse an opportunity to review the resident's care plan with the nursing assistant, the resident, the family, and/or the legal representative.

Residents often become more anxious when they are restrained and fight against the restraint (Wykle, 1991). If the nurse notices that the resident has become agitated, confused, or fearful, he or she may assign an appropriate staff member to remain with the resident until the resident is calm and comfortable. The length of time for the staff member to remain with the resident varies depending on each resident's individual response to being restrained.

Three cases that illustrate how to apply these principles in different situations deserve special mention here. The first concerns initial application of a restraint to a resident who is behaving violently. Because at least two staff members are needed to protect the resident from injury, a nurse should help the nursing assistant apply the restraints. The nurse may also need to request additional help while applying the restraint to ensure the safety of other residents as well as that of staff members (Sorrentino, 1992). The resident may also need a sedative if his or her violent behavior does not cease after the restraint has been applied.

The second case involves initial application of a restraint to a resident who is cognitively impaired. Two staff members should apply the restraint. Because a resident who is cognitively impaired may be unable to understand why he or she is being restrained, the presence of a second staff member can help to divert the resident's attention while the restraint is being applied as well as soothe and comfort the resident afterward.

The third case concerns the resident who needs a restraint to keep his or her body aligned properly when sitting. Usually, a physical or occupational therapist, clinical nurse specialist, or restorative care nurse will have been present to help the nursing staff try out various devices that promote proper body alignment before they apply the restraint (American Health Care Association, 1990). When the time comes to apply the restraint, the same therapist or nurse may wish to be present again to make sure that the device fits properly and that other staff members know how to use it. Some positioning devices are complex pieces of equipment that are individually constructed, or molded, to fit a resident's individual body shape. When such complicated positioning devices are used as physical restraints, it is essential to follow three recommendations:

1. Provide thorough training for all staff members who will use the device before they actually apply it.

2. Display the device's user instructions in a highly visible location for the convenience and safety of the resident, the family member or legal representative, and the staff (see Table 7.1).

3. Make sure that either the device's sales representative or the appropriate staff therapist or nurse is on call for at least 24–48 hours after the device is applied to answer staff members' questions or address their concerns.

Physician Order A physician order usually is required whenever a restraint is used (American Health Care Association, 1990; Ohio Department of Health, 1988; Sorrentino, 1992). Generally, this order describes the specific type of restraint, the reason for using the restraint, the frequency and duration of use for the restraint, and the schedule of release periods for exercise (Rose, 1987). An example of such an order for a vest restraint might read as follows:

> Soft vest restraint, to be used every day, in chair or in bed, to prevent resident from abusing self or other residents during an episode of violent behavior. Release restraint when resident is calm. Total time in restraint is not to exceed 1 hour per use. Notify MD if resident is not calm within 1 hour or if resident has three violent episodes in 24-hour period.

Staff members should also know and follow both the facility's own policy and the state's laws for long-term care facilities regarding additional requirements for restraint orders. For example, Ohio regulations require that the attending physician examine the resident personally before authorizing the use of physical restraints in any nonemergency situation (Ohio Department of Health, 1988).

Care During Period of Restraint

Observation Throughout the time that a physical restraint is used, staff members are required to observe and assess the resident frequently to ensure his or her physical and psychosocial well-being. The use of a restraint never replaces the need for staff observation; rather, it increases the amount of observation that the resident needs. The frequency of monitoring periods reported in the literature varies from every 15 minutes to every 2 hours (Darby, 1990; Kendrick & Wilber, 1986; Mezey & Lynaugh, 1991; Roper, Coutts, Sather,

& Taylor, 1985; Wiest, 1990). Some residents may need continuous monitoring, whereas others may require checks at 30-minute intervals. A professional nurse should establish the frequency of monitoring after making a systematic assessment of the problem that led to restraint use and the resident's response to the application of the restraint. When monitoring the resident, the nursing assistant should observe the resident to determine the following:

1. Is the resident safe?
2. Is the resident's behavior changing in any way?
3. Is the resident comfortable?
4. Does the physical restraint place the resident's physical well being in jeopardy in any way such as from skin irritation, restricted circulation to limbs, or restricted breathing secondary to tightness of the restraint?

The nursing assistant may also offer the resident psychological support and reassurance during the times when the facility's social worker is not available to do so.

In addition to the nursing assistant's frequent observations, regular assessment by a professional nurse is required. In discussing physical restraint and seclusion for psychiatric patients, Roper and colleagues (1985) recommend hourly assessments, whereas McCoy and Garritson (1983) prefer assessments every 2 hours. In the long-term care setting, both Morrison and colleagues (1987) and Rose (1987) recommend assessing the resident at least every 8 hours to determine whether the physical restraint needs to be continued. Rose also states that hourly assessments are necessary when restraints are used that severely restrict a resident's movement, such as bilateral wrist and ankle restraints. Hence, the frequency of assessments clearly depends on three key elements:

1. The resident's condition and response to the restraint
2. The type of restraint
3. The reason for using the restraint

Because physical restraints deprive residents of their freedom, documentation of care is essential. Documentation of monitoring and assessment data provides critical information that the interdisciplinary team must have to evaluate the resident's need for ongoing use of the restraint (American Health Care Association, 1990; American Nurses Association, 1987; Calfee, 1988; Fulmer et al., 1983; Kendrick & Wilber, 1986; McCoy & Garritson, 1983; Morrison et al., 1987; Roper et al., 1985; Sorrentino, 1992; U.S. Food and Drug Administration, 1991). Table 7.2 presents a list of the information that should be documented in the resident's record.

Maintenance of Physical Function   The goal of nursing care for residents in long-term care facilities is to help the resident attain and maintain the highest level of physical, mental, and psychosocial well-being that is practical for him or her (American Health Care Association, 1990). Physical restraints severely restrict a person's ability to move, and in some cases, may completely immobilize a resident. Many studies have demonstrated the serious consequences of excessive or prolonged restraint use and immobilization for older adults (Blakeslee, Goldman, Papougenis, & Torell, 1991; Brower, 1991; Evans & Strumpf, 1989; Evans et al., 1991; Miller, 1975; Rader & Donius, 1991; Schwartz, 1990; Strumpf & Evans, 1988; Tadsen & Brandt, 1973; Wiest, 1990).

The caregiver can help prevent residents from suffering many of the negative effects of immobilization. Nursing care interventions to help achieve this include:

1. Permitting the resident, if able, to meet his or her own needs (e.g., performing basic care tasks, walking, taking care of personal hygiene, using the toilet, and eating and drinking) or helping the resident do these things

2. Encouraging the resident to maintain an active range of motion in his or her limbs, or exercising the person's limbs passively

3. Providing the resident's bed or chair with the appropriate pressure-relieving devices during the period of restraint

4. Restraining the resident in positions that protect him or her from possible asphyxiation

5. Repositioning the resident to check his or her circulation and loosening the restraints to prevent skin irritation at least every 1–2 hours, or more frequently if problems occur or if the resident's condition warrants

6. Using the least restrictive physical restraint possible

While a resident is restrained, staff should monitor and record carefully both fluid intake and urinary output to prevent the resident from becoming dehydrated. Residents who can drink fluids by themselves should have water within easy reach, or staff should offer fluids every time they check the resident.

When a resident is unable to exercise, the caregiver can help maintain the person's flexibility by performing passive range of motion exercises on the person's limbs. Because an older adult's skin is thin, fragile, and easily injured, the caregiver should remove one re-

Table 7.2.   Documentation requirements for restrained residents

- Note any incident in which a patient or resident slips out of his or her restraint, charting it immediately after reapplying the restraint.
- Record observations of the patient's or resident's level of consciousness, activity level, color, general appearance, hydration level, amount of perspiration, and skin temperature.
- Explain why the patient or resident is being restrained. Describe the type of restraint being used.
- Document any discussion with the patient or resident, his or her physician, or the person's family about the need for restraint.
- Note any decision by the patient or resident or his or her family about using the restraint.
- Note the frequency with which the restraint is checked, removed, and reassessed to ensure the patient's or resident's safety, comfort, and freedom.
- Describe the way the restraint fits. (Proper fit minimizes the risk of trauma from the restraint, which can increase, rather than decrease, the patient's or resident's agitation.)
- Consult another nurse or manager about the need for restraint if a patient or resident refuses to consent to use of the restraint, documenting the reasons for using the restraint and asking the nurse or manager to co-sign the note.

Adapted from Calfee (1988).

straint at a time carefully during the exercise period to prevent skin tears or abrasions that may result when the restraint pulls or rubs against the resident's skin. The caregiver should also observe the skin condition of the entire limb carefully, noting particularly the color and condition of the skin directly under the restraint and inspecting pressure points for any redness. The resident who wears wrist and/or ankle restraints may need to have protective padding wrapped around the limb before the restraint is applied to prevent skin injury. This padding must be changed frequently and should be well secured so as to keep the resident from slipping out of the restraint. The caregiver should remove a resident's mitt restraints when exercising the fingers and wrists, cleansing the hands, cutting the nails, and observing the color and condition of the skin. A hand roll may be used to keep the hand in a natural position.

Some restraints are secured in place with knotted cloth straps, whereas others may have a locking device that opens only with a combination lock or a key. So that the resident in such a restraint may be released quickly in an emergency, all nursing staff should carry the key or written combination with them at all times. Keys or written combinations may also be posted in a clearly visible location that is close to the restrained resident (Sorrentino, 1992). For the residents whose restraints are secured with knotted cloth straps, the staff should place a pair of scissors nearby (but out of the resident's reach) so that they can cut off the restraints quickly in an emergency (Sorrentino, 1992).

Residents who are restrained in geri-chairs or any other type of chair from which they cannot rise easily by themselves require special attention. Staff must ensure that such residents' needs for skin care, fluids, regular visits to the toilet, and exercise are addressed. Caregivers should reposition residents who are restrained and provide some form of exercise, such as walking, every hour. Residents with skin problems should be repositioned even more frequently.

Most importantly, the entire team must set a realistic limit on the amount of time the restraint may be left in place before the resident is given a rest period from it. Milne (1988) recommends that a resident should be restrained for no more than 8 hours without being released, and that the resident should remain free for at least another 8 hours before any further physical restraint is applied. Setting such a standard encourages the care team to seek innovative alternatives to restraints.

Maintenance of Psychosocial Function Maintaining a resident's psychosocial functioning is as important as maintaining his or her physical functioning. The staff should make every effort to ensure the restrained person's privacy. Being restrained is a dehumanizing experience (Matteson & McConnell, 1988). Residents may cry out in despair, screaming, "I don't know why they would want to tie me up like this!" or "Please, don't do this!" (Rose, 1987, p. 20). Anger, discomfort, resistance, demoralization, and fear of abandonment are some of the feelings expressed by residents who are restrained (Evans & Strumpf, 1989; Rose, 1987; Strumpf & Evans, 1988). Moreover, the restraint itself may place a resident in a dangerous situation. For example, because the resident is immobilized, agitated, and crying out for help, other residents who are annoyed by the noise may abuse the person, either physically or verbally. Alternatively, other residents may feel saddened by the restrained resident's cries and attempt to help by untying the restraints.

Coordination of interventions and cooperation among the various team members are essential if a resident is to regain and maintain his or her highest level of psychosocial functioning. Interventions to enhance the restrained resident's self-esteem may require the help of family members, social workers, recreational therapists, nurses, or nursing assistants. Residents who are anxious may benefit from receiving an explanation of why they must be restrained and from having someone remain with them to provide emotional support until their anxiety subsides. The team will also need to plan interventions for residents who become distressed by the emotions that the restrained residents display. Nursing staff, too, may need supportive interventions and opportunities to vent their feelings about having to restrain a resident.

Accurate documentation of the resident's mental status and behavioral response to physical restraints is vital. Kendrick and Wilber (1986) have developed a flow chart that provides a comprehensive view of the resident's behavior over an 8-hour period "to ease the crucial task of recording the staff's frequent interventions and checks of patient behavior" (p. 1117). A similar flow chart could be developed to document the frequent monitoring and assessment data, the restorative interventions implemented to maintain the restrained resident's optimal physical and psychosocial function, and evaluation of the effectiveness of the restraints in achieving the desired outcomes of care for the resident. Table 7.2 presents a list of information that should be documented on a flow chart.

EVALUATION

During the period of restraint, the nursing staff and other members of the interdisciplinary team must continually evaluate the effectiveness of the physical restraint in achieving the desired outcome of care. Evaluation determines whether or not the intervention has helped the resident and whether or not the reason for using the restraint still exists. When a resident's restraints are removed, the staff should talk with the resident about the experience, if the resident is cognitively able. Because the experience of being restrained is frightening, the resident will need reassurance both after the restraints are applied and after they are removed.

The mission of the care facility's quality assurance committee is to provide ongoing evaluation of three main issues: 1) the effectiveness of the interdisciplinary team in maintaining a restorative care environment in which restraint use is limited; 2) the effectiveness of physical restraints in correcting or resolving residents' problems when other, less restrictive alternatives fail; and 3) the safety of residents who are physically restrained. With feedback from the quality assurance committee on these issues, the team is better able to initiate creative alternatives to restraint use and is more likely to use physical restraints only as a last resort.

CONCLUSION

"Caring societies must protect the freedom of vulnerable individuals from excessive restrictions, cruel and unusual punishment and invasion of privacy" (Robbins, 1986, as quoted in Evans & Strumpf, 1989, p. 70). The success of maintaining a restorative care environment depends upon the interdisciplinary team's creative problem-solving abilities and collaborative efforts to ensure that the facility's residents are free from excessive restrictions. The team must view physical restraints as potentially dangerous, strictly temporary measures that are used rarely, and then only as a last resort. The care team that follows the guidelines for safe use of physical restraints and the standards of restorative care is most likely to help its residents preserve their dignity and attain their highest possible level of functioning.

REFERENCES

American Health Care Association. (1990). *The long term care survey: Regulations, forms, procedures, guidelines.* Washington, DC: Author.

American Nurses Association. (1987). *Standards and scope of gerontological nursing practice.* Kansas City, Missouri: Author.

Blakeslee, J.A., Goldman, B.D., Papougenis, D., & Torell, C.A. (1991). Making the transition to restraint-free care. *Journal of Gerontological Nursing, 17*(2), 4–8.

Brower, H.T. (1991). The alternatives to restraints. *Journal of Gerontological Nursing, 17*(2), 18–22.

Calfee, B.E. (1988). Are you restraining your patients' rights? *Nursing, 18*(5), 148–149.

Darby, S.J. (1990). Containing the wanderer. *Nursing Times, 86*(15), 42–43.

Evans, L.K., & Strumpf, N.E. (1989). Tying down the elderly: A review of the literature on physical restraint. *Journal of the American Geriatrics Society, 37*(1), 65–74.

Evans, L.K., Strumpf, N.E., & Williams, C. (1991). Redefining a standard of care for frail older people: Alternatives to routine physical restraint. In P.R. Katz, R.L. Kane, & M.D. Mezey (Eds.), *Advances in long-term care* (Vol.2, pp. 81–108). New York: Springer-Verlag.

Fulmer, T., Dix, G., Yoder, A., & Terrill, J. (1983). Nursing guidelines for the use of restraints in nonpsychiatric settings. *Journal of Gerontological Nursing, 9*(3), 180–181.

Gordon, M. (1987). *Nursing diagnosis: Process and application* (2nd ed.). New York: McGraw-Hill.

Katz, L., Weber, F., & Dodge, P. (1981). Patient restraint and safety vests: Minimizing the hazards. *Dimensions in Health Service, 58*, 10–11.

Kaufmann, M.M. (1991, April). Initiating a restraint reduction program in a nursing home. In C. Dunn (Moderator), *Restraint reduction in long-term care—Cleveland models.* Symposium conducted at the Ninth Annual Florence Cellar Conference of Gerontological Nursing, Cleveland, OH.

Kaufmann, M.M. (in press). Activities in the nursing home setting. In B. Bonder (Ed.), *Functional performance in the elderly.* Philadelphia: F.A. Davis.

Kendrick, D.W., & Wilber, G. (1986). When in seclusion. *American Journal of Nursing, 86*(10), 1117.

Matteson, M.A., & McConnell, E.S. (1988). *Gerontological nursing: Concepts and practice.* Philadelphia: W.B. Saunders.

McCoy, S.M., & Garritson, S. (1983). Seclusion: The process of intervening. *Journal of Psychosocial Nursing and Mental Health Services, 21*(8), 9–15.

Mezey, M., & Lynaugh, J. (1991). Teaching nursing home program: A lesson in quality. *Geriatric Nursing, 12*(2), 76–77.

Miller, M. (1975). Iatrogenic and nursigenic effects of prolonged immobilization of the ill aged. *Journal of the American Geriatrics Society, 23*, 360–369.

Milne, C. (1988). Using restraint. *Nursing Standard, 2*(36), 24.

Morrison, J., Crinklaw-Wiancko, D., King, D., Thibeault, S., & Wells, D.L. (1987). Formulating a restraint use policy. *Journal of Nursing Administration, 17*(3), 39–42.

Ohio Department of Health. (1988). *Nursing and rest home law and rule.* Columbus, OH: Author.

Rader, J., & Donius, M. (1991). Restraints in the '90s: Leveling off restraints. *Geriatric Nursing, 12*(2), 71–73.

Robbins, L.J. (1986). Restraining the elderly patient. *Clinics in Geriatric Medicine, 2*(3), 591–599.

Roper, J.M., Coutts, A., Sather, J., & Taylor, R. (1985). Restraint and seclusion. *Journal of Psychosocial Nursing and Mental Health Services, 23*(6), 18–23.

Rose, J. (1987). When the care plan says restrain. *Geriatric Nursing, 8*(1), 20–21.

Schwartz, D. (1990). The use of physical restraints for the elderly. *Imprint, 37*(4), 54–57.

Sorrentino, S.A. (1992). *Textbook for nursing assistants* (3rd ed.). St. Louis: C.V. Mosby.

Stilwell, E.M. (1988). From the editor: Use of physical restraints on older adults. *Journal of Gerontological Nursing, 14*(6), 42–43.

Strumpf, N.E., & Evans, L.K. (1988). Physical restraint of the hospitalized elderly: Perceptions of patients and nurses. *Nursing Research, 37*(3), 132–137.

Strumpf, N.E., & Evans, L.K. (1991). The ethical problems of prolonged physical restraint. *Journal of Gerontological Nursing, 17*(2), 27–30.

Tadsen, J., & Brandt, R.W. (1973). Rules for restraints: Hygiene and humanity. *Modern Nursing Home, 30*, 57–58.

U.S. Food and Drug Administration. (1991). Potential hazards with protective restraint devices. *FDA Medical Bulletin, 21*(3), 3–4.

Wiest, M. (1990). The dilemma of using physical restraints. *Rehabilitation Nursing, 15*(5), 267–268.

Wolanin, M.O., & Phillips, L.R.F. (1981). *Confusion: Prevention and care.* St. Louis: C.V. Mosby.

Wykle, M. (1991). Physical restraints and the geropsychiatric patient. *Journal of Gerontological Nursing, 17*(2), 1.

Appendix 7.A

Sample Philosophy of Nursing Care

Margaret Wagner House of The Benjamin Rose Institute,
Cleveland Heights, Ohio

The activities of all nurses and nursing assistants employed by Margaret Wagner House are based on the fundamental philosophy of service to the elderly, and the promotion of learning and research. Individual contributions are coordinated and planned for the professional, scientific, and humanitarian care of residents. Whether the aim be preventive, maintenance, rehabilitative, or comfort, care is ultimately directed toward an optimum state of health.

The Nursing Services Department is dedicated to comprehensive nursing care that considers the physical, emotional, psychosocial, cultural, and spiritual needs of the individual older resident. In order to achieve this ideal, nurses work cooperatively in an interdisciplinary team effort to assess, plan, deliver, and evaluate care.

The Department strives to maintain an environment which recognizes and encourages individual effort and achievement, promotes learning, and stimulates the development of new ideas. The Department believes that staff development is an important part of providing such an environment. Nursing services personnel are provided opportunities to learn new skills and to broaden their gerontological nursing knowledge within both Margaret Wagner House and the community.

In the interest of contributing to the development of the field of Gerontological Nursing, the Department offers learning opportunities to nursing students at all levels and actively supports, conducts, and participates in research endeavors.

Appendix 7.B

Sample Policy
on Use of Physical Restraints

Margaret Wagner House of The Benjamin Rose Institute,
Cleveland Heights, Ohio

GENERAL PHILOSOPHY OF PHYSICAL RESTRAINT USE

Margaret Wagner House has a philosophy of not using physical restraints if at all possible. The use of physical restraints is discouraged at all times in the home. Restraints are to be used only as a last resort after other, less restrictive alternatives have been explored. Physical restraints may be used on residents only in *special cases* or in *emergency situations*. Consent to use restraints must be obtained from resident and/or family/legal representative. Consent must be documented in Resident's Clinical Records.

1. General policy
   a. Physical restraints are not to be used on residents except in SPECIAL CASES or EMERGENCY SITUATIONS when other alternatives have been explored and the safety and welfare of a resident require a restraint. Preferably, the decision to implement physical restraints is made by the interdisciplinary team whenever possible. Any use of physical restraints must be approved by the Assistant Director of Nursing. The only exception is an *emergency situation*.

   b. Any orders for restraints under the situations specified below must be in writing by the physician and must be specific as to type of restraints, reasons for restraints, and duration of restraints. All restraints will be released at least every two (2) hours and the resident exercised and/or ambulated.

   c. Efforts will subsequently continue to reduce the time the resident is required to be in the physical restraint or to eliminate the restraint altogether.

Source: From the sample policy of Margaret Wagner House of The Benjamin Rose Institute, Cleveland Heights, OH. Copyright © 1992, Margaret Wagner House; reprinted by permission.

    d. The Head Nurse/designee will evaluate the effectiveness of the physical restraint in the monthly summary.

2. Emergency situations

    a. An *emergency situation* is defined as protecting a resident from injury to self or those around him/her.

    b. This may include residents becoming extremely aggressive, destructive, or violent.

    c. In cases of emergency, residents may only be restrained for a period not exceeding twelve (12) hours without notification to the Assistant Director of Nursing.

    d. An order must be obtained by the Head Nurse/Charge Nurse from the Physician.

    e. The Nursing Supervisor is immediately informed of the emergency and the application of restraints.

3. Special cases
The use of a physical restraint will be allowed only if the family/legal representative or resident absolutely insists on its use; or, if different alternatives to physical restraint prove to be unsuccessful on a particular resident. The charge nurse on the unit will be responsible for informing the Assistant Director of Nursing/Supervisor of such situations. The Head Nurse/Social Worker/Assistant Director of Nursing/Supervisor will continue to educate the family/legal representative and/or resident to try alternatives to restraints. Should such efforts fail, permission will be given by the Director of Nursing or the Assistant Director of Nursing. The Head Nurse/Charge Nurse will call a physician to obtain a written order. Subsequently, this information will be documented on the Monthly Indicator List.

4. In both *special cases* and *emergency situations*, the use of physical restraints will be monitored and reviewed by the Head Nurse/Interdisciplinary Team (IDT)/Assistant Director of Nursing.

    a. Head Nurse—monthly summary

    b. IDT—quarterly review at Resident Care Conference

    c. Assistant Director of Nursing—monthly via Indicator List

    d. An order for a physical restraint must be reviewed and signed by the attending physician every thirty (30) days.
A monthly list of bed/chair restrained residents will be submitted to the Assistant Director of Nursing by the Unit Coordinator on the first of every month.

5. Admissions to the home will be informed by Social Services during the admission process of the general philosophy of care on physical restraint use.

6. PT and OT will be available for consultation regarding alternatives for physical restraints, especially when the resident has a positional problem.

7. Therapeutic Recreation will plan individual/group activities for the resident to facilitate the reduction/elimination of the physical restraint.

8. The Education Department will annually inservice all staff on the Philosophy of Restraint Reduction and Alternative to Restraints.

9. The Interdisciplinary Team consists of the Resident, Family/Legal Guardian, Medical Director, Director of Nursing or designee, Head Nurse, Nursing Assistant, Therapists (PT/OT), Therapeutic Recreation, Social Services, Pharmacist, and Dietitian.

Chapter 8

Physical Restraints in the Hospital Setting

Lorraine C. Mion and J. Dermot Frengley

INCIDENCE OF PHYSICAL RESTRAINT USE IN THE HOSPITAL SETTING

Several studies have examined the incidence of physical restraint use among nonpsychiatric hospitalized patients. In the general acute care setting, about 6%–17% of patients had been restrained at some time (Frengley & Mion, 1986; Lofgren, MacPherson, Granieri, Myllenbeck, & Sprafka, 1989; Mion, Frengley, Jakovcic, & Marino, 1989; Robbins, Boyko, Lane, Cooper, & Jahnigen, 1987). However, among patients over 65, the range increases to 18%–20.3%; among patients 75 and older, the figure rises to 22% (Frengley & Mion, 1986; Mion, Frengley, & Adams, 1986; Robbins et al., 1987; Warshaw et al., 1982). Thus, one of every five older adult patients on a general medical or surgical unit will be restrained at some time.

FACTORS DETERMINING WHO IS RESTRAINED

Two studies have examined some of the factors that determine whether or not a patient is likely to be physically restrained in the acute care setting (Mion, Frengley, et al., 1989; Robbins et al., 1987). The severity of the patient's illness, the presence of cognitive and/or physical impairments, and the diagnosis of presence of a psychiatric condition increase the patient's risk of being physically restrained by a factor of at least four in the acute medical setting (Mion, Frengley, et al., 1989). In addition, Robbins and colleagues (1987) found that medical and surgical patients' risk of being physically restrained increased at least threefold if they were impaired cogni-

127

tively, had undergone surgery, or needed devices used to treat an underlying medical disorder that restricted their mobility (e.g., intravenous lines). Hence it appears that regardless of age, patients who reveal impaired cognition, poor judgment, or behavior disorders together with impaired physical function are most likely to be physically restrained.

ACTUAL AND PERCEIVED BENEFITS OF RESTRAINING HOSPITAL PATIENTS

One of the main reasons for restraining older patients in nonpsychiatric settings is to ensure their safety by keeping them from falling. If physical restraints truly were effective, one would expect them to prevent falls. Yet, 13%–47% of older patients who fall are physically restrained (Colling & Park, 1983; Gross, Shimamoto, Rose, & Frank, 1990; Lund & Sheafor, 1985; Mion, Gregor, et al., 1989; Walshe & Rosen, 1979; Wieman & Ovear, 1986). The value of physical restraints is thus questionable. No clinical trials have tested the effectiveness of physical restraint as an intervention to prevent falls. However, one study of older patients in a 160-bed geriatric department of an 850-bed teaching hospital gathered data on the effectiveness of restraints before and after the implementation of a policy limiting physical restraint use (Powell, Mitchell-Pedersen, Fingerote, & Edmund, 1989). The researchers reported the number of falls for the 2 years preceding the implementation, the year of the implementation itself, and the 4 years following it. Although the rate of falls increased slightly, no change occurred in the rate of falls that resulted in injury. Thus, there is little or no evidence that restraints prevent fall injury or that removing them causes fall injury (Powell et al., 1989).

A second possible benefit of using physical restraints is the sense of security that some patients may feel because of the presence of the restraint (Hoaglund, 1991). Patients' psychological responses to physical restraints vary, however, and the caregiver must examine this issue thoroughly with each patient.

ADVERSE EFFECTS ASSOCIATED WITH RESTRAINING HOSPITAL PATIENTS

Many complications have been reported as a direct result of the use of a physical restraint, but these have not been well studied. The most serious complication is death caused by strangulation from the physical restraint. Reports of 15 deaths have appeared in the medical literature, and a review by Fried cites 30 such occurrences (DiMaio,

Dana, & Bux, 1986; Dube & Mitchell, 1986; Fried, 1987; Hunt, 1990; Katz, Weber, & Dodge, 1981; Staff, 1990). Among the severe or permanent complications that have been reported are nerve injuries, joint contractures, and shortage of oxygen to the brain resulting from strangulation by the restraint (Berrol, 1988; McLardy-Smith, Burge, & Watson, 1986; Miller, 1975; Scott & Gross, 1989; Yob, 1988).

Mild-to-moderate or short-term complications, such as hyperthermia and new bladder or bowel incontinence, have also been reported (Lofgren et al., 1989; Mclardy-Smith et al., 1986; Miller, 1975). In the only prospective study on mild-to-moderate physical complications (Lofgren et al., 1989), 102 consecutively restrained patients in an acute medical service of a Veterans Administration hospital were observed from admission to discharge. The researchers found that the longer the patient was physically restrained, the greater was the rate at which new pressure sores and hospital-acquired infections developed.

Other adverse effects of physical restraints are psychological distress and significantly decreased social activity. Studies have shown that from one-fifth to one-half of older adults suffer psychological distress as a result of being physically restrained and that as many as one-third of restrained older patients suffer significantly reduced social activity (Folmar & Wilson, 1989; Mion, Frengley, et al., 1989; Strumpf & Evans, 1988; Tinetti, Liu, Marottoli, & Ginter, 1991).

The number of hospital deaths is significantly higher among restrained patients than among nonrestrained patients in similar age groups (Frengley & Mion, 1986; Mion, Frengley, et al., 1989; Robbins et al., 1987). The fact that older adults who are restrained suffer more severe illnesses and higher mortality rates than do those who are not restrained may call into question our present standard of care of older adults in acute care wards.

MAKING DECISIONS ABOUT PHYSICAL RESTRAINTS

Nurses are usually the primary decision makers regarding the use of physical restraints. Although physical restraints require a physician's order, in most cases, nursing staff initiate their use without such an order (MacPherson, Lofgren, Granieri, & Myllenbeck, 1990; Mion, Frengley, et al., 1989). Several studies have examined the many reasons that hospital nurses give for using restraints on specific patients. By far the most common reason is to keep the patient from falling. According to surveys of nurses, approximately 60%–77% of restrained patients were put in restraints to keep them from falling; 34%–40% to keep them from disrupting therapies; 19%–23% to keep them from wandering, 11%–18% to manage behavioral problems; and 11% to help them maintain their posture (MacPherson et al., 1990; Mion, Frengley, et al., 1989; Strumpf & Evans, 1988).

The caregiver has no clear indicators to use as guidelines for when and why a patient should be physically restrained. Different nurses will give different reasons for using physical restraints on the same patient (MacPherson et al., 1990; Mion, Frengley, et al., 1989; Yarmesch & Sheafor, 1984). Nurses differ among themselves, and nurses and physicians disagree with one another (MacPherson et al., 1990). The lack of agreement among health care providers on when and why patients should be restrained adds to the controversy surrounding this practice.

ALTERNATIVES TO PHYSICAL RESTRAINTS

Because rationales for physical restraint use vary, no single approach is likely to be effective as an alternative method of care. Rather, a variety of approaches that involve the staff, the physical environment, and the patient will likely be the most effective way to deal with the patient in the acute care setting. The sections that follow examine some of the challenges that caregivers face when dealing with older hospital patients and the alternatives that can help them avoid using restraints.

Alternatives for Preventing Falls

Preventing falls is the most common reason nurses give for using physical restraints in the general hospital setting. Older adults often fall, and when they do, they may sustain serious injury, such as fracture. Older people fall for a variety of interacting reasons. Caregivers must carefully evaluate the reasons why a particular patient is at risk of falling so that interventions can be tailored to address the specific risk factors facing the individual patient. In addition, caregivers must evaluate the environmental factors that can contribute to falls. Environmental factors include not only the architectural characteristics of the hospital setting, but staff characteristics as well (Hogue, 1984). For example, several hospital-based studies have shown that the largest proportion of falls occurs during times when the largest number of staff are on duty (Mion, Gregor, et al., 1989; Morse, Tylko, & Dixon, 1987; Sehested & Severin-Nielsen, 1977). In this case, the availability of staff rather than their numbers appears to correlate with peak fall times (Morse et al., 1987). Hence, implementing fall prevention programs means examining both unit- and facility-wide policies.

Table 8.1 lists some of the most common factors associated with falls among older patients. Environmental factors often can be eliminated or altered by the staff. Individual factors vary in kind and degree from patient to patient, and will determine the approaches used for each individual patient. Table 8.2 provides an overview of staffing, environmental, and patient-centered interventions to prevent falls. The sections that follow describe specific interventions to prevent falls.

Interventions for Dealing with Poor Balance and Posture Control
Patients who have poor muscle strength in the trunk frequently have trouble maintaining an upright sitting position. These patients may have been restrained to keep their posture upright and to keep them from sliding or falling out of the chair. Alternative interventions are aimed at improving the person's sitting balance via modifications to furniture or props. Most hospital chairs are straight-backed chairs whose seat and backrest form approximately a 90° angle. Reclining chairs or wheelchairs that have a 70°–75° angle with a modified leg lift can help keep the patient's center of gravity in the chair seat while maintaining the patient's upright position. Consulting with an occupational therapist is often helpful, since he or she may be able to suggest material, cushions, or other props that help keep the patient upright while preventing him or her from sliding out of the chair. For example, Dycem™ is a thin, waterproof material that occupational therapists commonly place under a stroke patient's dinner plate to prevent the plate from sliding across the table. Used on

Table 8.1.   Factors that contribute to patient falls in the hospital setting

Physical factors	Environmental factors
Visual or perceptual problems	Obstacles
Musculoskeletal and gait disorders	Clutter
Stroke	Furniture
Parkinson's disease	Elevated beds
Arthritis	Chairs on wheels
Foot problems	Bedside tables on wheels
Confusion	Glare
Low blood pressure upon standing	Diminished lighting
Dizziness	Wet or slippery floors
Weakness	Improper or ill-fitting footwear
Poor balance or postural control	
Blood pressure medications	
Psychotropic drugs	
Narcotic analgesics	
Cardiac arrhythmias	
Fainting	

Table 8.2. Strategies for preventing falls in the hospital

Staffing strategies	Environmental strategies	Patient-centered strategies
Examine falls within setting	Clear pathways of hazards and potential hazards	Rehabilitate to improve strength and balance
Examine organizational factors that contribute to falls	Install safety features (grab bars, signal buttons with extended cords)	Provide physical aids (walking, visual, hearing)
Restructure staff routines to increase number of available staff throughout day	Modify furniture (lower bed heights, keep bedside drawers within easy reach)	Modify clothing (skid-proof shoes, flat heels, robes no longer than ankle length)
Set and maintain toilet schedules as ongoing policy	Provide adequate lighting, especially in bathroom at night	Use devices to maintain posture or balance in chair (Dycem™ to prevent sliding)
Install electronic alarms	Install carpeting in bathrooms	
	Consult occupational and/or physical therapist	

the patient's chair seat or chair cushion, this material will prevent the patient from slipping out of the chair. Wedge cushions inserted with the narrower side into the back of the chair seat can also be used to keep the patient from slipping out of the chair. Bolster cushions may be used to lift the patient's trunk into an upright position rather than allowing him or her to slump forward or to the side.

Interventions for Dealing with Weakened or Impaired Gait
The older patient whose gait is weakened or impaired is at risk of falling for different reasons and hence needs a different set of interventions. Often, acute medical or surgical conditions in older adults can be direct causes of weakened or impaired gait. For patients who were able to live independently before they were hospitalized, helping them to walk as soon as possible is especially important to avoid the negative effects of immobility (Hirsch, Sommers, Olsen, Muller, & Winograd, 1990; Reddy, 1986). A decline in a patient's level of functioning can also mean discharge to a nursing home rather than a return home (Hirsch et al., 1990). Hence, nursing staff should remain alert to the risk of diminished function among their older adult patients.

A restorative care approach may be instituted early in the patient's hospital stay. For example, when patients do not require complete bedrest, allowing them to walk to the toilet with supervision or assistance rather than use the bedpan helps prevent disability from disuse and also maintains muscle strength (Reddy, 1986). As endurance improves, the level of exercise can be increased (e.g., assisted walking can be done several times a day). Several articles published by nurse clinicians are available that describe successful formal exercise programs for older hospital patients (Milde, 1988; Paillard & Nowak, 1985; Warnick, 1985). Consultation with a physical therapist can help the caregiver decide whether the patient needs assistive devices as well as individualized activity plans.

Patients with weakened or impaired gait may be at risk of falling when trying to get in or out of bed. The bed should be high enough to allow the patient's feet to touch the floor comfortably while he or she is sitting on the bed. Hospital beds typically are too high for older adults, especially if pressure-relieving devices are placed on top of the mattress. One way to lower the bed is to have the maintenance department replace the bed's wheels with wheels of a smaller diameter. In addition to the problems it poses for the safe transfer of patients, bed height can also interfere with the patient's sensory perceptions (Wolanin & Phillips, 1981). Even with the head of the bed inclined, a patient in a hospital bed cannot see the angle at which the walls meet the floor, and so cannot judge accurately how far it is from the edge of the bed to the floor.

The older patient who has both weakened or impaired gait and impaired cognition poses additional challenges for the nursing staff. These patients should be helped to walk early in their hospital stays. However, because of their cognitive impairments, these patients need to be observed especially carefully. This can be done in several ways. Moving the patient closer to the nurses' station, shortening the intervals between nurses' rounds (e.g., making rounds every half hour instead of every hour), and starting a routine toilet schedule are measures that help ensure that staff members have ample opportunities to observe their patients. Enlisting the help of family members, especially early in a patient's hospitalization, is often useful, particularly during the second or third shifts, when fewer staff members are on duty. Hospital volunteers can also help monitor patients. Finally, a variety of electronic alarms, described in Table 8.3, are available to monitor patients. Typically, early sounding alarms (such as weight-sensitive and tension-trigger alarms) are needed for patients who are physically and cognitively impaired and are likely

Table 8.3. Electronic alarms available for monitoring hospital patients

- Sophisticated video monitors
- Weight-sensitive devices for beds or chairs that sound an alarm when the patient shifts his or her weight off the device
- Devices that attach to the bedframe or chair back on one end and to the patient on the other so that tension on a pulled string or cord sounds an alarm
- Devices that attach to the patient's legs and sound an alarm when the patient's body position changes
- Devices that attach to the patient and sound an alarm only when the patient exits through a doorway

to fall. If funds are not available for electronic alarms, the signal button cord can be pinned to the patient's gown so that a warning signal goes off when the patient attempts to leave the bed or chair.

Alternatives for Protecting or Maintaining Medical Therapy

The second most common reason for restraining older hospital patients is to protect or maintain the routes or devices used to provide therapy. Here, too, caregivers must be creative and thoughtful in rethinking how best to provide the patient's medical care.

The first question to ask is whether the patient truly requires the device that the staff wants to protect. Intravenous (IV) lines and indwelling urinary catheters, followed by nasogastric tubes, are the most common devices that caregivers try to maintain or protect (MacPherson et al., 1990). Interestingly, MacPherson and associates (1990) found that physicians tended to recommend use of physical restraints to protect devices that they were solely responsible for restarting or reinserting, whereas nurses tended to protect devices that they were responsible for restarting or reinserting. These findings raise concerns that physical restraints may be used, in part, for staff convenience.

A second question is whether the removal or disruption of the device is life threatening and whether the patient is likely to suffer immediate harm. Clearly, the disruption of an indwelling urinary catheter should be treated differently from the disruption of a ventilator. Both the nurse and the physician must weigh the potential benefits of using the restraint against the potential risks associated with immobilizing the patient.

If a patient does need a particular route or device, the caregiver must then determine whether alternative methods of delivery can be used to avoid having to use the physical restraint. For example, if a urinary catheter is medically necessary, can intermittent straight catheterization be used instead of a long-term indwelling catheter? Does the patient require an intravenous route for medication, or can a different route be used? If the patient is able to drink sufficient amounts of fluid, can a Heplock rather than a continuous infusion IV line be used to deliver medication? Nurses and physicians working closely together can devise alternative care plans that place the patient first and the equipment second.

Any medical device will feel strange to the older patient. In all cases, giving the patient a simple explanation of the device and allowing him or her to feel the device while a caregiver closely watches may reassure the patient, thus decreasing the chance that the patient may remove it. If the device is absolutely necessary for the patient's well-being and nursing staff believe that the patient is likely to disrupt the therapy, several alternative strategies, as detailed below, can still be tried before resorting to wrist restraints.

Interventions for Protecting Intravenous Sites Covering or camouflaging the insertion site may be enough to keep a confused patient from disrupting the intravenous line. This can be accomplished by using Kerlix® gauze or Kling® wrap, Thera-Band® arm casings (used for burn patients), or long-sleeved hospital gowns or robes. The IV pole and bag should be kept behind the patient and out of his or her visual field. If keeping the IV out of sight is not enough to deter the patient from actively pulling the line out, mitts (semi-firm hand enclosures that keep the fingers extended) or foam finger extenders (usually obtained through the occupational therapy department) should be tried. These devices allow freedom of arm movement but prevent patients from being able to grasp the IV line. Mitts or hand rolls that flex the fingers should not be used since they can cause loss of function.

Interventions for Maintaining Nasogastric Tubes Nasogastric tubes used for suction can be hard to maintain in a confused older adult. The insertion site cannot be camouflaged and usually the person feels some discomfort from the tube itself. The caregiver should give the patient simple, consistent explanations. If restraints are necessary, the less restrictive ones, such as mitts or foam finger extenders on both hands, should be tried first. Many times, a confused and sick patient is cognitively and physically unable to coordinate his or her hand and arm movements well enough to grasp the tube. In this case, the patient will be able to bat at the tube but not dislodge it. If a wrist restraint is ultimately necessary, the caregiver might limit the restraint to only one of the patient's arms while using mitts or foam finger extenders on both hands.

If nasogastric tubes are used for feeding, it may be possible to find alternative routes. Feeding tubes may be placed early in the course of the illness if the patient has a diminished level of consciousness, impaired swallowing, and/or weakened or absent gag and cough reflexes. At frequent intervals throughout the patient's hospital stay, the caregiver should reevaluate the patient's ability to swallow in order to ensure that the feeding tube is not left in place unnecessarily. Speech and occupational therapists should be consulted in handling patients with nasogastric tubes.

If the patient needs long-term tube feeding, the caregiver might consider placing a percutaneous endoscopic gastrostomy tube (PEG). The insertion site heals easily once the PEG is removed. Because it is relatively easy to camouflage the PEG with clothing, abdominal dressings, and abdominal binders, a confused patient may not need wrist restraints.

Interventions for Maintaining Urinary Catheters Patients who are admitted to acute medical and surgical units from the emergency room frequently have indwelling catheters in place. As with the nasogastric tube, the caregiver should first decide whether the catheter is medically necessary. If it is, a straight catheter routine might be considered as an acceptable alternative. If the indwelling catheter is medically necessary and the straight catheter routine is unacceptable, the caregiver might still try restrictive mitts or foam extenders before resorting to wrist restraints. The catheter should always be removed as soon as is medically feasible to reduce the patient's risk of hospital-acquired infection or developing new urinary incontinence.

Alternatives for Managing Wandering

A patient who wanders usually has a high level of physical mobility but has cognitive impairments that interfere with his or her ability to stay oriented to place. The staff's primary concerns are to keep the person from falling by removing any environmental hazards, to prevent his or her exposure to inclement weather, and to prevent pedestrian accidents (Fopma-Loy, 1988).

Wandering may be either aimless or purposive. The caregiver's interventions will differ depending upon the patient's type of wandering, as shown in the following sections.

Interventions for Managing Aimless Wandering The patient who wanders aimlessly paces without apparent purpose or destination. This is the patient who walks in and out of other patients' rooms, has a short attention span, and is easily distracted. Patients who wander typically have significant cognitive impairments that affect their orientation, memory, and ability to socialize (Snyder, Rupprecht, Pyrek, Brekhus, & Moss, 1978). Wandering has been explained in various ways, and it may reflect some facet of the patient's previous lifestyle, extreme restlessness, or a need for more stimulation (Fopma-Loy, 1988; Snyder et al., 1978). Interventions for the patient who wanders should focus on maintaining a safe environment while allowing the person freedom of movement (Heim, 1986).

The caregiver must carefully assess the patient's physical status and ability to walk. If the patient's gait is weak or impaired, the interventions described earlier in this chapter should be instituted. Assessment should focus on the patient's actual behavior. Does the patient wander only at certain times of the day or following certain events? The family can provide valuable input about the history and description of their relative's behavior, and the caregiver can make note of any interventions that have been successful.

Once the assessment has been completed, the environmental interventions may begin. Hospital corridors are frequently cluttered with equipment, laundry bags, and other items, especially during the busy times of patient care. Keeping one side of the hallway free of equipment or obstacles at all times helps ensure that the older patient has a safe walkway. The caregiver should also assess the patient's room for potential obstacles, such as footstools. Adequate lighting at night and the use of partial rather than full siderails will help ensure that the patient can get to the toilet easily. The patient's footwear should also be considered. If the hospital slippers fit poorly, the nursing staff may want to ask the family to bring the patient's shoes or slippers from home.

A major concern of staff is the patient who tries to leave the unit without the staff's knowledge, especially if stairwells are nearby. If the unit is not equipped with electronic buzzers, then empty soft drink cans or a small hand-held dinner bell may be tied to the frame of an exit door to warn staff that a patient is trying to leave. Staff members who work the night shift find this strategy especially helpful.

If a patient needs frequent observations, he or she may be moved closer to the nurses' station, and all personnel on the floor should be alerted that the patient may tend to wander. Taping a card with the patient's name and unit number to the back of his or her clothing alerts staff in other areas of the hospital that the patient is on the wrong floor. Establishing a regular toileting schedule also helps keep the patient from wandering, especially at night.

Visual cues can be used to help orient the patient as well as to help keep him or her from leaving the floor. A sign with the patient's first name printed in large boldface letters may be placed outside the patient's room. Strategically located chairs near the nurses' station or beside open doorways, for example, may help divert the patient, who then sits down instead of leaving the unit.

Sometimes the strategic placement of movable screens or furniture is enough to keep the patient within a defined space or room. Cloth or plastic strips secured across the doorway at waist height may be enough to keep a patient within his or her own room. Some researchers have also reported that patients who get regular physical exercise wander less frequently than do sedentary patients (Fopma-Loy, 1988). Hence, planned periods of walking may help reduce the person's tendency to wander.

Communication between the caregiver and the patient must be clear and goal oriented. Directions that are kept simple and are stated positively are more likely to be followed than those that are phrased negatively (Rader, 1987). For example, a patient will under- . stand "Walk over here" much more easily than "Don't go out the door." Using a negatively phrased command requires the patient to think of the concept first and then to avoid carrying through the action suggested by the concept (Rader, 1987).

Interventions for Managing Purposive Wandering Purposive behavior is usually more difficult to manage than aimless wandering, since patients who wander purposefully usually are agitated or have coexisting behavioral problems. The patient who wanders purposefully does so with a specific goal or objective (Snyder et al., 1978). The patient may be seeking a specific task or job to do or may be looking for a person or place (Snyder et al., 1978). For example, the patient may insist that he or she must get to the store before it closes. An older woman may insist upon seeing her children, whom she remembers as being very young and in need of her care, even though they are now middle-age adults. Patients who wander purposefully are more challenging to deal with because they actively want to leave the floor and are harder to distract than are those who wander aimlessly.

Simple diversions or manipulations of the environment are not generally successful with patients who wander purposefully. Rader, Doan, and Schwab (1985, 1987) have systematically studied and implemented a variety of approaches to deal with wandering patients, whom they call "exit-seekers." Many of their approaches can be adapted to the acute care setting, since most involve hospital personnel.

Early identification of the patient as potentially having a tendency to wander is essential to implementing a structured, consistent approach. Caregivers on all three shifts of this patient's unit must communicate with each other to establish a clear sense of teamwork and a consistent care plan (Rader, 1987; Rader et al., 1985).

Rader uses the term *agenda behavior* to describe the actions of a patient who wanders purposefully (1985, 1987). The term refers not only to the patient's actions, but also to the emotional needs that underlie those actions. Rader and associates (1985, 1987) have found that focusing on the patient's emotions or underlying needs is by far the most effective means of dealing with someone who purposefully wanders. Thus, in dealing with a patient who believes that she must return home in order to take care of her children, staff should acknowledge the woman's underlying needs. They then might try to distract her by asking her about her family and what she enjoyed doing with her children. This approach sometimes helps lessen the patient's need to leave.

If the patient insists upon leaving the floor, he or she should be allowed to do so only if his or her medical status so permits and if accompanied by a staff member. A patient who has grown tired and who has become aware of being disoriented usually will agree to return to his or her own room to rest if a staff member suggests it.

It is essential that staff members learn how to phrase and voice their suggestions when dealing with patients who wander purposefully. Attempts to orient such patients to reality often merely increase their anger or agitation. These patients are sensitive to the caregiver's nonverbal behavior and tone of voice. Any gesture or nuance that the patient interprets as corrective or argumentative will increase his or her desire to leave the unit.

Table 8.4 lists some possible interventions for both aimless and purposive wandering. Whenever possible, it is best to avoid restraining the patient who wanders. Immobilizing such a person increases his or her agitation (Werner, Cohen-Mansfield, Braun, & Marx, 1989) and frequently leads to the concomitant use of psychotropic drugs to control the person's induced agitation.

Alternatives to Managing Agitation and Disruptive Behavior

Physical restraints sometimes are used to manage behaviors that are seen as disruptive, such as those that occur with delirium tremens. In older patients, disruptive behavior may result from delirium or from chronic dementia. Since agitation or disruptive behaviors that result from acute delirium are self-limiting, this section of the chapter focuses on the agitation and disruptive behaviors that accompany dementia.

To the older patient, being admitted to the hospital is a fright-

Table 8.4. Strategies for managing aimless and purposive wandering in the hospital

Staffing strategies	Environmental strategies	Patient-centered strategies
Use same staff person consistently.	Camouflage doorways and exits.[a]	Participate in planned physical activity.
Enlist help of family, volunteers, and other patients in monitoring patient's movements.	Install cloth or plastic strips across doorways.[a]	Participate in diversionary activities.[b]
Remain nonthreatening and avoid confrontation.	Use visual cues.[a]	
	Create safe "pacing routes."[a]	
Avoid use of negatives.	Modify room assignments.	
Keep requests simple.	Install exit alarms.	
Distract and redirect.		

[a]Applies to aimless wandering only.
[b]Applies to purposive wandering only.

ening and anxiety-provoking event. The patient who suffers from dementia cannot process the multitude of stimuli, and his or her symptoms may appear to worsen rapidly. A common example is the patient who experiences a so-called "catastrophic reaction," or overreaction to a benign stimulus. This is the patient whose emotions erupt or who lashes out during a simple procedure such as a blood pressure reading or a bath.

Interventions for Preventing Agitation and Disruptive Behavior Prevention of agitation or disruptive behavior is considerably easier than management of such behavior. Caregivers should thus create an environment that is least likely to cause the patient to become agitated. Families of patients who are known to have dementia should become involved in shaping their relative's care plan as early as possible. Because the presence of a familiar loved one helps to reassure the confused patient, visiting hours should be relaxed. It may also help to have a family member present during the night. Small personal objects brought from home may also help make the environment seem more familiar to the confused patient. Both family members and primary caregivers are valuable sources of information regarding the patient's typical behavior, the events or situations that provoke catastrophic reactions in the patient, and the warning signs or behaviors that can alert staff to watch for the patient's impending catastrophic reaction. If the patient's agitated behavior is repetitive or predictable, interventions may be aimed at preventing its occurrence. One such intervention would be the judicious use of a small dose of an anxiolytic drug before the time at which the patient's predictable reaction occurs.

The number of personnel who care for the patient should be limited. When the same staff members consistently provide the patient's care, the patient may come to recognize his or her caregivers. As the environment begins to seem more familiar, the patient's anxiety eases. Using the same caregiver consistently also enhances the primary nurse's ability to evaluate the patient's behavior accurately.

Agitation and disruptive behavior are common in people with Alzheimer's disease. The sleep–wake cycle may be altered in such patients because of the disease process; hospital routines can exacerbate sleep disturbances. The unit's routines should be modified as necessary to give the older patient as many undisturbed hours at night as possible. For example, if the patient must receive medications at night, it is best to arrange for all of them to be given simultaneously, so that the patient is awakened only once. The goal of not disturbing the patient's sleep more than is absolutely necessary should also be kept in mind in terms of monitoring vital signs. If the patient's condition is stable, the middle-of-the-night reading may be eliminated, or it may be taken when the patient must be awakened for medication or another procedure.

Because a patient with Alzheimer's disease is easily overwhelmed, staff members should try to reduce the number of stimuli present in the patient's immediate environment. At the same time, they must take care not to deprive the person of sensory stimulation.

Reducing noise in the hospital environment has been advocated for patients of all ages, not just for confused older adults (Topf, 1984; Williams, 1988). Excessive noise annoys patients, increases their heart rate, and disturbs their sleep patterns (Topf, 1984; Williams, 1988). The noise from three or four adjoining bedrooms with competing televisions, radios, telephones, intercoms, and conversation can be overwhelming for patients with Alzheimer's disease. Television can be particularly stressful if the patient believes that the people or events that appear on television are real. Family members or caregivers will know whether television causes the patient to become anxious or agitated. Caregivers should answer the patient's call light in person, and avoid, whenever possible, using the intercom to page other staff members. Where a patient with Alzheimer's disease has been assigned a room that is particularly noisy, caregivers should try to move the patient to a quieter room.

Excessive or inadequate illumination may increase the patient's discomfort or anxiety. The patient should have enough light to see clearly what is in the room but not so much that it disrupts his or her sleep. Because the patient with Alzheimer's disease cannot always identify the causes of his or her discomfort, the caregiver should also monitor the room temperature. Feeling too hot or too cold may also trigger disruptive behavior.

Communication, both verbal and nonverbal, with the person with Alzheimer's disease is very important. Even though the patient may be unable to communicate, he or she remains sensitive to the speaker's tone of voice. The caregiver should convey calmness and friendliness, and should never rush a patient with Alzheimer's disease. Instructions should be kept clear and simple, and all actions should be explained to the patient, since people with Alzheimer's disease may interpret simple acts, such as taking a temperature, as acts of aggression.

Interventions for Managing Agitation and Disruptive Behavior
Once a patient has become agitated or disruptive, nursing interventions should be aimed at calming the patient down. In general, patients with Alzheimer's disease are not assaultive. Typically, such patients become combative or strike out only when it appears to them that others are trying to harm them. People with Alzheimer's disease rarely initiate action. Therefore, caregivers should take a different approach from that used with a truly violent or assaultive person. First, the caregiver must reduce the number of stimuli to which the patient is subjected. This means turning off the radio or television and keeping the number of people in the room to a minimum. The caregiver should also stay within the patient's visual field. Approaching the patient from the back or side may startle the person and provoke him or her into striking out in fright. The caregiver's tone of voice should remain friendly and conversational. This may be difficult to accomplish if the patient still can speak fluently and is verbally abusive. However, maintaining one's verbal composure is important, since patients with Alzheimer's mimic others. Nonverbal behavior must also remain nonthreatening. Caregivers should maintain eye contact when speaking with patients, and should keep their own arms down along the sides of the body so that the confused patient does not interpret the caregiver's posture as threatening. The caregiver should never argue with or try to explain to a distraught, confused patient, since the patient will interpret the attempt as corrective or argumentative, and may thus escalate his or her own disruptive behavior. Sometimes strategies such as simple diversion or focusing on the patient's feelings can help reduce the patient's agita-

tion. If the caregiver is the focus of the patient's anger, he or she should leave the room and allow another staff member to sympathize with the patient, reassure him or her, and thus diffuse the patient's anger and agitation. Typically, when the first caregiver returns later in the shift, the patient with Alzheimer's disease will not remember the incident.

Physically restraining an already agitated patient increases the person's anxiety and agitation. Psychotropic drugs do not work quickly in older patients whose emotions are already out of control, and the drugs' tranquilizing effect may not become evident for several hours. The caregiver should first try all other means to calm the patient and diffuse the situation before resorting to physical restraints or psychotropic drugs.

CONCLUSION

Reducing the use of physical restraints in acute care settings is best accomplished by increasing the staff's awareness and knowledge of alternative methods of care (Frengley & Mion, 1989). Caregivers need not feel alone in caring for older adults. Professionals in other health care disciplines are valuable allies and the members of the interdisciplinary team should be involved in choosing the alternatives to physical restraints.

REFERENCES

Berrol, S. (1988). Risks of restraints in head injury. *Archives of Physical Medicine and Rehabilitation, 69*, 537–538.

Colling, J., & Park, D. (1983). Home, safe home. *Journal of Gerontological Nursing, 9*, 175–179, 192.

DiMaio, V.J.M, Dana, S.E., & Bux, R.C. (1986). Deaths caused by restraint vests. *Journal of the American Medical Association, 255*, 905.

Dube, A.H., & Mitchell, E.K. (1986). Accidental strangulation from vest restraints. *Journal of the American Medical Association, 256*, 2725–2726.

Folmar, S., & Wilson, H. (1989). Social behavior and physical restraints. *Gerontologist, 29*, 650–653.

Fopma-Loy, J. (1988). Wandering: Causes, consequences, and care. *Journal of Psychiatric Nursing and Mental Health Issues, 26*(5), 8–18.

Frengley, J.D., & Mion, L. (1989). Physical restraint in acute hospitals. In L. Evans & N. Strumpf (Chairs), *Routine physical restraint: Historical context and re-examination of the practice in hospitals and nursing homes.* Symposium conducted at the 42nd Annual Meeting of the Gerontological Society of America, Minneapolis, Minnesota.

Frengley, J.D., & Mion, L.C. (1986). Incidence of physical restraints on acute general medical wards. *Journal of the American Geriatrics Society, 34*, 565–568.

Fried, J. (1987, June 21). Care that kills. *Long Beach Press-Telegram* [California] (pp. C4–C5).

Greenland, P., & Southwick, W.H. (1978). Hyperthermia associated with chlorpromazine and full-sheet restraint. *American Journal of Psychiatry, 135*, 1234–1235.

Gross, Y.T., Shimamoto, Y., Rose, C.L., & Frank, B. (1990). Why do they fall? Monitoring risk factors in nursing homes. *Journal of Gerontological Nursing, 16*, 20–25.

Heim, K.M. (1986). Wandering behavior. *Journal of Gerontological Nursing, 12*(11), 4–7.

Hirsch, C.H., Sommers, L., Olsen, A., Muller, L., & Winograd, C.H. (1990). The natural history of functional morbidity in hospitalized older patients. *Journal of the American Geriatrics Society, 38*, 1296–1303.

Hoaglund, E. (1991). Restraint myths? Or facts? [Letter]. *Geriatric Nursing, 12*, 12.

Hogue, C.C. (1984). Falls and mobility in late life: An ecological model. *Journal of the American Geriatrics Society, 32*, 858–861.

Hunt, A.R. (1990). Legal issues involved in the use of restraints: Analyzing the risks. In *Untie the elderly: Quality care without restraints* (Serial No. 101-H, pp. 28–32, 203–209). Washington, DC: U.S. Government Printing Office.

Katz, L., Weber, F., & Dodge, P. (1981). Patient restraint and safety vests: Minimizing the hazards. *Dimensions in Health Services, 58*, 10–11.

Lofgren, R.P., MacPherson, D.S., Granieri, R., Myllenbeck, S., & Sprafka, J.M. (1989). Mechanical restraints on the medical wards: Are protective devices safe? *American Journal of Public Health, 79*, 735–738.

Lund, C., & Sheafor, M.L. (1985). Is your patient about to fall? *Journal of Gerontological Nursing, 11*, 37–41.

MacPherson, D.S., Lofgren, R.P., Granieri, R., & Myllenbeck S. (1990). Deciding to restrain medical patients. *Journal of the American Geriatrics Society, 38*, 516–520.

McLardy-Smith, P., Burge, P.D., & Watson, N.A. (1986). Ischaemic contracture of the intrinsic muscles of the hands: A hazard of physical restraint. *Journal of Hand Surgery, 11*, 65–67.

Milde, F.K. (1988). Impaired physical mobility. *Journal of Gerontological Nursing, 14*(3), 20–24.

Miller, M.B. (1975). Iatrogenic and nursigenic effects of prolonged immobilization of the ill aged. *Journal of the American Geriatrics Society, 23*, 949–956.

Mion, L., Frengley, J.D., & Adams, M. (1986). Nursing patients 75 years and older. *Nursing Management, 17*, 24–28.

Mion, L.C., Frengley, J.D., Jakovcic, C.A., & Marino, J.A. (1989). A further exploration of the use of physical restraints in hospitalized patients. *Journal of the American Geriatrics Society, 37*, 949–956.

Mion, L.C., Gregor, S., Buettner, M., Chwirchak, D., Lee, O., & Paras, W. (1989). Falls in the rehabilitation setting: Incidence and characteristics. *Rehabilitation Nursing, 14*, 17–22.

Morse, J.M., Tylko, S.J., & Dixon, H.A. (1987). Characteristics of the fall-prone patient. *Gerontologist, 27*, 516–522.

Paillard, M., & Nowak, K.B. (1985). Use exercise to help older adults. *Journal of Gerontological Nursing, 11*(7), 36–39.

Powell, C., Mitchell-Pedersen, L., Fingerote, E., & Edmund, L. (1989). Freedom from restraint: Consequences of reducing physical restraints in the management of the elderly. *Canadian Medical Association Journal, 141,* 561–564.

Rader, J. (1987). A comprehensive staff approach to problem wandering. *Gerontologist, 27,* 756–760.

Rader, J., Doan, J., & Schwab, M. (1985). How to decrease wandering, a form of agenda behavior. *Geriatric Nursing, 6,* 196–199.

Reddy, M.P. (1986). A guide to early mobilization of bedridden elderly. *Geriatrics, 41*(9), 59–60, 63–64, 66–67, 70.

Robbins, L.J., Boyko, E., Lane, J., Cooper, D., & Jahnigen, D.W. (1987). Binding the elderly: A prospective study of the use of mechanical restraints in an acute care hospital. *Journal of the American Geriatrics Society, 35,* 290–296.

Rose, J. (1987). When the care plan says restrain. *Geriatric Nursing, 8,* 20–21.

Scott, T.F., & Gross, J.A. (1989). Brachial plexus injury due to vest restraints. *New England Journal of Medicine, 320,* 598.

Sehested, P., & Severin-Nielsen, T. (1977). Falls by hospitalized elderly patients: Causes, prevention. *Geriatrics, 32,* 101–108.

Snyder, L.H., Rupprecht, P., Pyrek, J., Brekhus, S., & Moss, T. (1978). Wandering. *Gerontologist, 18,* 272–280.

Staff. (1990). $39 million awarded in death. *American Journal of Nursing, 90,* 22.

Strumpf, N.E., & Evans, L.E. (1988). Physical restraint of the hospitalized elderly: Perceptions of the patients and nurses. *Nursing Research, 37,* 132–137.

Tinetti, M.E., Liu, W., Marottoli, R.A., & Ginter, S.F. (1991). Mechanical restraint use among residents of skilled nursing facilities. *Journal of the American Medical Association, 265,* 468–471.

Topf, M. (1984). A framework for research on aversive physical aspects of the environment. *Research in Nursing and Health, 7,* 35–42.

Walshe, A., & Rosen, H. (1979). A study of patient falls from bed. *Journal of Nursing Administration, 9,* 31–35.

Warnick, M.A. (1985). Acute care patients can stay active. *Journal of Gerontological Nursing, 11*(12), 31–35.

Warshaw, G., Moore, J., Friedman, S., Currie, E., Kennie, D., Kane, W., & Mears, P. (1982). Functional disability in the hospitalized elderly. *Journal of the American Medical Association, 248,* 847–850.

Werner, P., Cohen-Mansfield, J., Braun, J., & Marx, M.S. (1989). Physical restraints and agitation in nursing home residents. *Journal of the American Geriatrics Society, 37,* 1122–1126.

Wieman, H.M., & Ovear, M.E. (1986). Falls and restraint use in a skilled nursing facility. *Journal of the American Geriatrics Society, 34,* 907.

Williams, M.A. (1988). The physical environment and patient care. *Annual Review of Nursing Research, 6,* 61–84.

Wolanin, M.O., & Phillips, L.R.F. (1981). *Confusion: Prevention and care.* St. Louis: C.V. Mosby.

Yarmesch, M., & Sheafor, M. (1984). The decision to restrain. *Geriatric Nursing, 5,* 242–244.

Yob, M.O. (1988). Use of restraints: Too much or not enough? *Focus on Critical Care, 15,* 32–33.

Chapter 9

Outcomes of Removing Physical Restraints

Perla Werner and Jiska Cohen-Mansfield

On October 1, 1990, federal regulations implementing the Omnibus Budget Reconciliation Act of 1987 (OBRA '87) went into effect. These regulations state that a resident of a long-term care facility "has the right to be free from any physical restraints imposed or psychoactive drug administered for purposes of discipline or convenience and not required to treat the resident's medical symptom."

Caregivers have begun to implement these regulations, although with some reservation and apprehension. It is not easy to change an approach that is rooted in many years of practice, as is the use of restraints. However, changes in care had begun even before the regulations were implemented. Extensive discussions were held regarding the adverse physiological and psychological consequences associated with the use of physical restraints. These effects include pressure sores, decreased ability to socialize, urinary incontinence, increased agitation, psychological distress, and death by strangulation (Covert, Rodrigues, & Solomon, 1977; Frengley & Mion, 1986; Katz, Weber, & Dodge, 1981; Rosen & Giacomo, 1978; Werner, Cohen-Mansfield, Braun, & Marx, 1989).

Some institutions started to develop programs for reducing the use of physical restraints before the federal mandate. In response to state legislation requiring a reduction in the use of restraints, Florida's long-term care facilities reduced the number of residents who were restrained by half between August 1989 and March 1990 (Powills, 1990). In New Hampshire, educational workshops on restraint reduction started as early as February 1989, and more than 60 long-term care facilities reduced the use of restraints before the OBRA regulations were implemented (Rajecki, 1990). The long-term care system was ready for a change in philosophy and attitude, a change that the OBRA regulations legitimized.

Many recent conferences and articles have dealt with the topic of removing physical restraints (Werner & Cohen-Mansfield, 1991), and professionals continue to address questions concerning the implementation process. Alternatives to restraints are a matter of particular interest. This chapter examines the expected outcomes that this change in care brings to the care of frail older adults. Its finding are based on clinical impressions as well as empirical findings from several small studies of facilities that were pioneers in the removal of physical restraints. Several case studies are also presented as examples of successful implementation of a restraint removal program.

The outcomes presented in the case studies do not result merely from releasing a resident's physical restraints. Such outcomes may be expected only if a reduction in the use of physical restraints is accompanied by a complete change in the approach to care. Hence, nursing care should take a restorative care approach rather than a traditional custodial approach. The needs of nursing home residents should be evaluated by all the professionals and paraprofessionals involved in their care, including social workers, activities therapists, physical therapists, and others, and each resident should be treated according to an individualized care plan.

OUTCOMES FOR RESIDENTS

It is important to emphasize that immediate changes should not be expected when physical restraints are removed from a resident who has been restrained for a long time. Although the physical status of some residents may improve, it is likely that some physical capabilities may be permanently affected as a result of the neuromuscular deconditioning caused by a long period of immobility.

Falls and Injuries

The prevention of falls is one of the most frequently cited reasons for using physical restraints with a frail elderly resident. In a study of staff's perceptions of the use of physical restraints in the hospital, Strumpf and Evans (1988) found that the prevention of falls was the second most commonly cited reason by nurses (altered mental status was first). Despite this perception that restraints are effective in preventing falls, several studies have shown that physical restraints do not prevent falls (Lund & Sheafor, 1985; Tinetti, 1987; Walsh & Rosen, 1979; Werner et al., 1989). Moreover, removing physical restraints does not necessarily increase a person's likelihood of falling. A Canadian study of the removal of physical restraints in a hospital showed no clinically significant increase in the number of falls (Powell, Mitchell-Pedersen, Fingerote, & Edmund, 1989). Other facilities have also reported no change in the number of serious falls following the removal of physical restraints (Ejaz, 1991; Neufeld, Mulvihil, White, Brennan, & Libow, 1991). The clinical experience of staff at the Hebrew Home of Greater Washington shows that many residents who were initially restrained to keep them from falling deteriorated to the point where they were unable to move even without restraints. For these residents, physical restraints provide no benefit, and may be perceived as degrading and humiliating. Chapters 4, 5, and 6 of this volume examine the assessment of residents who may be at risk of falling and some of the alternatives for preventing falls that do not involve physical restraint.

Incontinence

A common physical consequence of prolonged immobilization is urinary incontinence (English, 1989), which usually occurs only a short time after the person is restrained. In a longitudinal study of 102 hospital patients whose average age was about 75 years, Lofgren, Richard, MacPherson, Granieri, Myllenbeck, & Sprafka (1989) found that 29% of the patients studied became incontinent of urine after an average of only 13.4 days. In addition to increasing a person's likelihood of becoming incontinent, physical restraints also make it more difficult for staff to offer the resident a consistent toilet schedule because of the additional effort involved in removing the resident's restraints. This, in turn, may result in other problems, such as pressure sores.

By reducing the use of physical restraints, caregivers may be able to prevent or delay the development of urinary incontinence in frail residents. Clinical experience shows that nursing staff find it easier to help a resident who is not restrained use the toilet, even though residents who have been restrained for a long time do not regain continence when their protective devices are removed. As a result, residents who are not restrained may have the opportunity to use the toilet more frequently, thus reducing complications such as pressure sores and dermatitis.

Agitation

For many years, physical restraints were the standard of care for agitated long-term care residents. Nursing staff restrained older adults to keep them from wandering, from hurting themselves or others, or from manifesting other agitated behaviors. Despite this widespread practice, many researchers have found that using physical restraints *increases* rather than decreases a resident's agitation (Blakeslee,

Goldman, Papougenis, & Torell, 1991; Gerdes, 1968; Werner et al., 1989). Reducing the use of physical restraints thus decreases the agitation that results from frustration over being restrained. It may also encourage staff members to develop creative and effective methods for managing agitation. These interventions may range from environmental safety measures to behavioral procedures for managing agitation. (For a thorough review of alternative methods for managing agitation, see Chapters 6 and 14 of this volume and Cohen-Mansfield, Werner, Marx, & Lipson [in press].)

Psychotropic Drugs

Many professionals have expressed concern that a reduction in the use of physical restraints will be accompanied by an increase in the use of chemical restraints. However, the OBRA regulations guard against this substitution. As early as 1982, when the Department of Geriatric Medicine at the St. Boniface General Hospital in Winnipeg decided to reduce its use of physical restraints, the staff also found that the use of psychotropic drugs decreased 26% in the 6 months evaluated, as compared with the same period the year before. Preliminary data from a study of the impact of the OBRA regulations on the use of physical and chemical restraints show that residents who had once been restrained were receiving significantly fewer antipsychotic drugs after their restraints were removed (Farley, Werner, Cohen-Mansfield, & Lipson, 1991).

Functional and Cognitive Ability

Although a resident's functional and cognitive abilities are not influenced directly by removing the physical restraints, they may be affected by a restraint-free policy. Residents who have been physically restrained for a long time are unlikely to become more cognitively intact or more functional simply because their restraints have been removed. In residents whose dementia is extreme, the deterioration caused by their prolonged immobility may cause them to become irreversibly dependent on caregivers to help them perform activities of daily living. However, a restraint-free policy is likely to prolong the functional independence of new residents. Because they remain more active, they are less likely to suffer from the physical deterioration or the sense of helplessness and loss of control that accompany the use of physical restraints.

Social Behavior, Participation in Activities, and Mood

One of the most often-cited effects of prolonged immobility in frail older adults is social withdrawal (Miller, 1975). In a study of 112 long-term care facility residents, Folmar and Wilson (1989) found that physical restraints hampered the residents' performance of social behavior. This, in turn, may cause the resident to become depressed and isolated. Therefore, one of the outcomes of removing a resident's physical restraints should be his or her increased participation in social activities. This increase is unlikely to be immediate and general. The effort to encourage residents' participation in activities should be a coordinated one, in which the activities therapist, other staff members, and family members define progressive goals for the resident based on his or her needs and limitations.

OUTCOMES FOR STAFF

The regulations concerning the removal of physical restraints have changed both nursing care for frail older adults and the role that staff members play when providing this care. To reduce the use of physical restraints, nursing care now must take a restorative, rather than a custodial, approach (see Chapter 5). When physical restraints are removed, some residents may be able to regain some of their physical abilities and become more independent in performing their activities of daily living, saving staff members' time and enabling the staff to socialize more often with the residents. Additionally, the need to develop creative, individualized alternatives to resident care encourages the staff to take a collaborative care approach. A multidisciplinary care team, which includes all professionals in the facility, such as social workers, activities therapists, physical therapists, and others, should discuss residents' needs and alternatives to restraints.

Several publications have addressed the guilt and distress that nursing staff members feel when they must restrain residents (McHutchion & Morse, 1989; Rose, 1987), as well as their fear of legal liability. Thanks to the OBRA regulations, nurses may no longer have to face many of the internal and external conflicts that occur when staff members must restrain an older person. This, in turn, may increase nursing staff members' satisfaction at work and minimize employee turnover in long-term care facilities.

OUTCOMES FOR FAMILIES

Family Participation

Family members' first reaction to the restraint reduction policy may be one of apprehension and distress. Concerned about the safety and well-being of their relatives, family members may be suspicious and are likely to put up some resistance. Staff members should meet with the family to explain and discuss the implementation of the new policy and to review the potential risks and benefits of alternative care options now available. Family members should be asked to describe any special needs of the resident and ways to enhance his or her care, such as playing a certain kind of music that may calm the resident. This information may help the staff develop creative alternatives to the use of physical restraints. Thus, because family members can play an active part in developing the care plan for the resident, restraint removal can become an opportunity to increase the family's participation.

Family Satisfaction

Many family members feel relieved that the resident is no longer restrained, and their satisfaction with the quality of care given their relative increases. The fears of those who felt apprehensive may be allayed after seeing that the resident has suffered no harm as a result of the new policy. Some relatives may remain concerned and fearful, however, especially if the resident falls. Staff should show special sensitivity toward these family members and should acknowledge their concerns, assuring them that if such an incident occurs, the staff will find out why the resident fell and set up a plan for preventing similar incidents in the future.

OUTCOMES FOR THE FACILITY

As with any other change, the introduction of a restraint removal program affects the entire facility. Administrators must become actively involved in the process and provide guidance and support to both staff members and families. Many administrators have expressed concern that the facility will need to hire more nursing staff as a result of the new policy. However, several studies show that facilities can reduce their use of physical restraints significantly without needing to increase the number of nursing staff (Mitchell-Pedersen, Fingerote, & Powell, 1985; Powell et al., 1989). The goal of restraint reduction may be attained by reallocating nursing time appropriately rather than by increasing the number of staff members. For example, nursing assistants who once devoted their time primarily to custodial care now may become involved in helping residents walk or in coordinating simple activity programs that help enhance the residents' social behavior (see Chapter 7).

Another concern that administrators frequently express involves the costs of implementing the new policies. However, clinical experience shows that costs are *lower* after a facility reduces the use of physical restraints, especially because of the savings on incontinence products (Powills, 1990).

The experience at the Hebrew Home of Greater Washington shows that it is possible to develop simple, effective alternatives without incurring major expenses (see Chapter 5). Additionally, because the new policy increases staff members' job satisfaction and thereby decreases the high staff turnover experienced in many long-term care facilities, the facility will likely save on the cost of training new employees.

CASE STUDIES

As the preceding sections have emphasized, most residents will not show an immediate change in their functional and cognitive status when their restraints are removed. With an appropriate restorative care approach, some residents may be able to recover some of the abilities they lost as a consequence of their prolonged immobilization. A facility that implements a restorative care philosophy may prevent or postpone the loss of residents' capabilities. Two case studies demonstrate the impact of this approach:

Ms. B., a 94-year-old widow, suffers from severe coronary artery disease, congestive heart failure, glaucoma, and osteoporosis. She entered the facility 2 years ago and was assigned to a light care unit. After approximately 1 year, Ms. B.'s cognitive ability began to deteriorate. She was diagnosed as suffering from Alzheimer's type dementia, and was transferred to a heavy care unit for residents with cognitive impairment. When transferred to her new unit, she became highly agitated and was restrained by means of a chair belt during the day shift and for 4 hours during the evening shift. While restrained, Ms. B. tried several times to get up, and fell.

After Ms. B. had been on the new unit for a short time, the rehabilitation nurse evaluated her and suggested removing her protective device and starting her on a regular walking program and toileting schedule. The staff informed Ms. B.'s family of these changes. Although they were hesitant and concerned about the possibility of her falling, they supported the new care plan.

Ms. B. started walking to lunch and dinner (a distance of 50 feet) with the assistance of a staff member. The goal of the walking program was to strengthen Ms. B.'s legs and to make walking a regular activity rather than an extraordinary effort. After 2 weeks in the walking program, Ms. B. started to walk independently, with the assistance of a walker. The new toileting schedule required that the nurses check Ms. B. hourly, and that they keep her close to the nurses' station when she was out of bed so that they could observe her closely.

Since Ms. B.'s restraints were removed 9 months ago, she has not fallen and she is no longer agitated. Ms. B. now participates in many structured activities and is in a good mood almost all the time. Staff members enjoy talking with her.

Ms. R., an 84-year-old widow, suffers from congestive heart failure, osteoporosis, and osteoarthritis. She entered the facility from the hospital 8 months ago after being treated for a hip fracture. When she entered the facility, she was bedridden and restrained by a posey vest. Although her cognitive ability is only moderately impaired, she has a serious problem communicating with staff because of her severely impaired hearing.

Shortly after her admission, the nursing rehabilitation consultant saw Ms. R. and initiated a walking program for her. Ms. R. was helped to walk 5 feet from her bed to the bathroom. After several days, she started to walk by herself at night, without supervision. Staff members were concerned that she might fall when she was unsupervised, and they consulted the rehabilitation nurse again. They solved this problem by placing a walker near Ms. R.'s bed at night and leaving her lights on. They also increased the amount of time and distance Ms. R. was to walk during the day.

Today, Ms. R. walks the full length of the corridor twice a day, and she no longer gets up at night. She communicates her needs to staff through gestures and signs. She gained 13 pounds in 8 months and she is very alert. Although staff tried several times to encourage her to participate in activities, she refused. As an alternative, a volunteer visits her regularly to provide her with one-to-one stimulation and recreation.

CONCLUSION

Reducing the use of physical restraints is an ongoing process. Everyone involved—nursing and other staff, residents, family members and administrators—should receive consistent support and reinforcement, as well as continuing education. Despite the immense progress that the new regulations have brought about, many aspects of restorative care still need to be explored:

- The effectiveness of different care alternatives to restraints needs to be studied, from clinical, safety, and financial points of view.
- Assessment tools are needed that have been developed for evaluating the individualized needs of residents systematically.

These instruments should guide caregivers in selecting better care practices for the resident being assessed.

* The perceptions and feelings of residents, families, and caregivers should be evaluated.

The removal of a resident's physical restraints may not result in obvious functional improvement. However, residents may feel a greater sense of dignity and self-respect and staff members may feel more satisfied with their work when caring for older adults without having to restrain them. The fact that removing physical restraints produces no adverse effects and provides the resident with more dignified care should be the most important reason for continuing the movement toward restraint-free care.

REFERENCES

Blakeslee, J.A., Goldman, B.D., Papougenis, D., & Torell, C.A. (1991). Making the transition to restraint-free care. *Journal of Gerontological Nursing,* *17*(2), 4–8.

Cohen-Mansfield, J., Werner, P., Marx, M.S., & Lipson, S. (in press). Assessment and management of behavior problems in the nursing home setting. In L.Z. Rubenstein & D. Wieland (Eds.), *Improving care in the nursing home (NH): Comprehensive reviews of clinical research.* Beverly Hills: Sage Publications.

Covert, A.B., Rodrigues, T., & Solomon, K. (1977). The use of mechanical and chemical restraints in nursing homes. *Journal of the American Geriatrics Society, 25,* 85.

Ejaz, F. (1991). *Evaluation of a program to reduce the use of physical restraints in two nursing homes in Cleveland.* Paper presented at the 44th annual scientific meeting of the Gerontological Society of America, San Francisco.

English, R.A. (1989, March). Implementing a non-restraint philosophy. *The Canadian Nurse, 85*(3), 293–300.

Farley, J., Werner, P., Cohen-Mansfield, J., & Lipson, S. (1991). *Psychotropic drug practice in the nursing home before and after the OBRA regulations: Description of an ongoing research.* Paper presented at the 22nd American Society of Consultant Pharmacists annual meeting, Montreal.

Folmar, S., & Wilson, H. (1989). Social behavior and physical restraints. *The Gerontologist,* *29*(5), 650–653.

Frengley, J.D., & Mion, L.C. (1986). Incidence of physical restraints on acute general medical wards. *Journal of the American Geriatrics Society, 34,* 565–568.

Gerdes, L. (1968). The confused or delirious patient. *American Journal of Nursing, 68,* 1228–1232.

Katz, L., Weber, F., & Dodge, P. (1981). Patient restraint and safety vests: Minimizing the hazards. *Dimensions Health Service, 58*(5), 10–11.

Lofgren, M.D., Richard, P., MacPherson, D.S., Granieri, R., Myllenbeck, S., & Sprafka, M. (1989). Mechanical restraints on the medical wards: Are protective devices safe? *American Journal of Public Health, 79*(6), 735–738.

Lund, C., & Sheafor, M.L. (1985). Is your patient about to fall? *Journal of Gerontological Nursing, 11*, 37–41.

McHutchion, E., & Morse, J. (1989). Releasing restraints: A nursing dilemma. *Journal of Gerontological Nursing, 15*(2), 16–21.

Miller, M.B. (1975). Iatrogenic and nursigenic effects of prolonged immobilization of the ill aged. *Journal of the American Geriatrics Society, 23*(8), 360–369.

Mitchell-Pedersen, L., Fingerote, E.L., & Powell, C. (1985). Let's untie the elderly. *Ontario Association of Homes for the Aged Quarterly, 21*(10), 10–14.

Neufeld, R., Mulvihil, M., White, H., Brennan, F., & Libow, L. (1991). *Effects of restraint removal on nursing home residents.* Paper presented at the 44th annual scientific meeting of the Gerontological Society of America, San Francisco.

Omnibus Budget Reconciliation Act of 1987. Public Law 100-203, Sections 4201(a), 4211(a).

Powell, C., Mitchell-Pedersen, L., Fingerote, E., & Edmund, L. (1989). Freedom from restraint: Consequences of reducing physical restraints in the managing of the elderly. *Canadian Medical Association Journal, 141*, 561–564.

Powills, S. (1990, July). More LTC facilities move to eliminate restraints. *McKnight's Long-Term Care Nursing,* 1.

Rajecki, R. (1990, January). Reducing restraint reliance. *Contemporary Long-Term Care,* 52–57.

Rose, J. (1987, January/February). When the care plan says restrain. *Geriatric Nursing,* 20–21.

Rosen, H.D., & Giacomo, J.N. (1978). The role of physical restraints in the treatment of psychiatric illness. *Journal of Clinical Psychiatry, 39*, 228–232.

Strumpf, N.E., & Evans, L.K. (1988). Physical restraints of the hospitalized elderly: Perceptions of patients and nurses. *Nursing Research, 37*(3), 132–137.

Tinetti, M. (1987). Factors associated with serious injury during falls by ambulatory nursing home residents. *Journal of the American Geriatrics Society, 35*, 644–648.

Walsh, A., & Rosen, H. (1979, May). A study of patient falls from bed. *Journal of Nursing Administrators,* 31–35.

Werner, P., & Cohen-Mansfield, J. (1991). *Reducing physical restraints in the nursing home: Clinical and research experiences.* Symposium presented at the 9th annual conference of the Maryland Gerontological Association, Baltimore.

Werner, P., Cohen-Mansfield, J., Braun, J., & Marx, M.S. (1989). Physical restraints and agitation in nursing home residents. *Journal of the American Geriatrics Society, 37*, 1122–1126.

Part III

Reducing the Use
of Chemical Restraints

Chapter 10

Chemical Restraints and the Proper Use of Psychotropic Drugs

Steven Lipson

This chapter examines the use of psychotropic drugs in long-term care facilities. In view of the federal regulations implementing the Omnibus Budget Reconciliation Act of 1987 (OBRA '87), which banned the use of psychotropic medications as restraints, it looks at appropriate and inappropriate ways in which such drugs can be used in long-term care facilities.

DEFINING CHEMICAL RESTRAINTS

Chemical restraints refer to any "psychoactive drug administered for purposes of discipline or convenience, and not required to treat the resident's medical symptoms" (Health Care Financing Administration, 1989). The use of chemical restraints with residents of long-term care facilities is prohibited by these federal regulations (42 C.F.R., part 481.13(a)).

USE OF CHEMICAL RESTRAINTS
IN LONG-TERM CARE FACILITIES

Since the 1970s, there have been repeated claims that the use of chemical restraints is routine in nursing homes. Two recent reports reveal that the practice continues. One study (Garrard et al., 1991) found that 50% of residents receiving antipsychotic drugs had no documented condition justifying their use. Another study (Johnson & DiBona, 1990) found that even when the resident's record documented that the choice of a psychotropic drug and the dosage were

159

appropriate for the resident's diagnosis and condition, the records contained no evidence that the resident had been monitored for therapeutic effect or side effects of the treatment.

Many cases of inappropriate drug use result from the mistaken belief that psychotropic drugs represent the only way of dealing with difficult behavior. Caregivers believe that the administration of drugs is helpful or benign, and do not perceive these actions as harmful or inconsistent with the maintenance of the resident's dignity and autonomy.

The following case study illustrates the sort of drug use that was once common and that is now prohibited by federal law:

Mrs. Miller, an 88-year-old widow, was living alone in the community with help from her family until she broke her hip 2 months before her admission to Pathwood Convalescent. During the postoperative period, she became confused and agitated at night. In the hospital, Mrs. Miller was started on a regular dose of 1 mg of haloperidol every day, and an order was given for an additional dose of 0.5 mg to be given every 6 hours as needed. These orders were continued when she was transferred to the nursing home for rehabilitation. The physical therapist found that Mrs. Miller was unable to cooperate in her therapy, and that she made little progress toward being able to walk independently. When Mrs. Miller's Medicare benefits were terminated because of her lack of progress, her family agreed that she should stay in the nursing home because of her "dementia."

The use of psychotropic drugs to treat Mrs. Miller would be considered a form of chemical restraint because her record contained no evidence of an assessment resulting in a diagnosis that required the use of a psychotropic agent. The drug-induced lethargy experienced by Mrs. Miller may, in fact, have contributed to her failure to make progress in regaining the ability to walk independently.

ASSESSING THE NEED FOR PSYCHOTROPIC MEDICATION

The intent of the federal regulations banning chemical restraint was to prevent facilities from using psychotropic drugs for purposes other than the treatment of psychiatric disorders. Where a psychiatric diagnosis is made, psychotropic drugs may be appropriate. Table 10.1 lists some of the specific conditions that may justify the use of some of the common antipsychotic agents listed in Table 10.2.

Diagnosing the more severe psychiatric disturbances, such as schizophrenia, psychotic mood disorder, or acute psychotic disor-

Table 10.1.   Specific conditions justifying use of antipsychotic drugs

1. Schizophrenia
2. Schizoaffective disorder
3. Delusional disorder
4. Psychotic mood disorders (including mania and depression with psychotic features)
5. Acute psychotic episodes
6. Brief reactive psychosis
7. Schizophreniform disorder
8. Atypical psychosis
9. Tourette's disorder
10. Huntington's disease
11. Organic mental syndromes (including dementia and delirium) with associated psychotic and/or agitated behaviors
    - Which have been quantitatively (number of episodes) and objectively (e.g., biting, kicking, scratching) documented
    - Which are not caused by preventable reasons, and
    - Which are causing the resident to
        - Present a danger to her/himself or to others,
        - *Continuously* cry, scream, yell, or pace if these specific behaviors cause an impairment in functional capacity, or
        - Experience psychotic symptoms (hallucinations, paranoia, delusions) not exhibited as dangerous behaviors or as crying, screaming, yelling, or pacing but which cause the resident distress or impairment in functional capacity, or
12. Short-term (7 days) symptomatic treatment of hiccups, nausea, vomiting, or pruritus.

Source: Health Care Financing Administration. (April, 1992). Interpretive guidelines. *State Operations Manual,* Transmittal 250.

ders, is generally not difficult. More attention needs to be paid to diagnosing less specific problems, such as agitation. The case study that follows illustrates the lack of care with which such problems are sometimes assessed and treated:

Mrs. Mark has just been admitted to the Maywood Nursing Home. Prior to entering the facility, she had lived alone in an apartment with part-time help from an aide. She was admitted to the facility after her aide and family noticed that she became agitated when she was asked to take a bath or get dressed.

Six months prior to entering the facility, Mrs. Mark's physician had prescribed a 0.5 mg of lorazepam three times a day. On the day of her admission to Maywood, she was disoriented and lethargic. In the evening, she became highly agitated, calling out continuously and striking the nursing assistants. Her physician ordered a dose of 1 mg of lorazepam.

To see how cavalierly drugs were prescribed in this case, imagine that Mrs. Mark's symptom had been fever instead of agitation. Although acetaminophen might have been administered to reduce her temperature, a cause of the fever would have been sought, a presumptive diagnosis made, and specific treatment given as appropriate. In this case, by way of contrast, no effort was made to determine why Mrs. Mark was agitated, or whether some underlying organic cause such as infection, a drug side effect, urinary retention, constipation, or pain may have been responsible for her disorientation. Rather than simply prescribe a psychotropic drug, the physician should have tried to determine the cause of Mrs. Mark's symptoms and then sought to treat them.

Assessment of the agitated resident can be difficult. Side effects of medication, physical conditions, and environmental factors all may contribute, as shown in the following sections.

Assessing the Side Effects of Medication

Medications often cause reversible confusion in frail older adults. Since virtually any class of therapeutic agent may be at fault, it may be difficult to determine which drug is responsible. Generally, the

Table 10.2. Commonly used antipsychotic drugs

Generic name	Brand name
acetophenazine	Tindal
chlorpromazine	Thorazine
chlorprothixene	Taractan
clozapine	Clozaril
fluphenazine	Prolixin, Permitil
haloperidol	Haldol
loxapine	Loxitane
mexoridazine	Serentil
molindone	Moban
perphenazine	Trilafon
prochlorperazine	Compazine
promazine	Sparine
trifluoperazine	Stelazine
triflupromazine	Vesprin
thioridazine	Mellaril
thiothixene	Navane

Source: Health Care Financing Administration. (April, 1992). Interpretive guidelines. State Operations Manual, Transmittal 250.

physician should look first for a recent change in dosage or the addition of a new medication. Medications that were started several weeks before the symptoms appeared may also be involved. In the case of Mrs. Mark, when her lorazepam was discontinued, her agitation decreased over a period of 2–3 days. Although her dementia remained and she still resisted some aspects of care, she was generally pleasant and compliant.

Assessing the Effect of Physical Conditions

Hearing or visual impairment may cause a resident to misunderstand a staff or family member and to be mislabeled as delusional. Serious conditions, such as hypotension, myocardial infarction, pneumonia, or stroke, may cause changes in behavior. Minor conditions, such as upper respiratory infection, constipation, or joint pain, may also affect behavior, particularly in frail residents in whom a change in behavior warrants a careful evaluation rather than the immediate administration of a psychotropic drug.

Assessing the Effect of Environmental Factors

Environmental factors may also play a role in agitation. A resident who complains that a stranger entered his room and tried to attack him may simply have been frightened by an unfamiliar nursing assistant who entered the room during the night in order to check on the resident. A move to a new room, a different seat in the dining room, a change in routine, or an unfamiliar face or picture on the wall may upset the resident's emotional equilibrium and result in a change in behavior or level of agitation.

Formal Psychological or Psychiatric Assessment

When the cause of a resident's problem remains unclear, psychological or psychiatric evaluation by a professional should be requested. The primary caregiver should ask the consultant to provide a complete diagnosis of the resident and specific recommendations for his or her care. Results of the evaluation should be shared with all staff members caring for the resident, and with the family if appropriate.

USE OF PSYCHOTROPIC AND OTHER DRUGS IN LONG-TERM CARE FACILITIES

Psychotropic drugs are used widely in long-term care facilities. Recent studies (Beers et al., 1988; Lantz, Louis, Lowenstein, & Kennedy, 1990; Sloane et al., 1991) have shown that about half of a facility's residents are receiving one or more psychotropic drugs. These drugs include antipsychotics, antidepressants, anxiolytics, sedatives, and hypnotics. The longer a resident remains in the facility, the more likely he or she is to be given such medications: among residents who have lived in the facility for 5 years or longer, 70% are on psychotropic drugs (Lantz et al., 1990).

Residents of long-term care facilities tend to be on many types of medications. A 1991 study found that the average resident takes 4.7 different medications a day (Sloane et al., 1991). Many of these drugs, including antihistamines, analgesics, antihypertensives, corticosteroids, and anticonvulsants, may affect their behavior. Although these drugs could also be used to control behavior, attention has focused on the use of psychotropic drugs—namely, antipsychotics, anxiolytics, antidepressants, sedatives, and hypnotics.

Psychotropic drugs are drugs used to treat mental illnesses. In the nursing home, they are most often used to treat problem behavior, anxiety, sleeping problems, and depression. An in-depth examination of the variety of psychotropic drugs available is beyond the scope of this chapter. (Readers are referred to recent publications such as Jenike [1989].) The sections that follow focus on a general approach to using psychotropic drugs.

Antipsychotic Drugs

Antipsychotic drugs are tranquilizers that are often used to treat residents whose behaviors are associated with certain organic mental syndromes, such as dementia. They are also used to treat psychotic disorders, such as schizophrenia and paranoia. The most commonly used antipsychotic drugs are listed in Table 10.2.

In recent years, the use of benzodiazepine tranquilizers in the nursing home has been discouraged. Residents who take these drugs tend to fall more frequently, and those with dementia become even more confused and lethargic, particularly when the longer-acting drugs, such as diazepam (Valium) and chlordiazepoxide (Librium), are used. These latter drugs should rarely, if ever, be used with nursing home residents. Even shorter-acting drugs, such as lorazepam (Ativan) and alprazolam (Xanax), should be used sparingly in the nursing home, since some of these drugs, particularly Xanax, can cause a physiological addiction, with severe and prolonged withdrawal symptoms when they are discontinued. In accord with the recommendations of Jenike (1989), the staff of the Hebrew Home of Greater Washington have found that small doses of thioridazine (Mellaril) and haloperidol (Haldol) are most effective in treating difficult behaviors in demented residents and produce the mildest side effects.

Anxiolytic Drugs

The benzodiazepine anxiolytics and some of the newer drugs, such as buspirone (Buspar), which causes little sedation, may be effective in residents with mild or no dementia who suffer from anxiety. In general, the physician should select the shorter-acting agents, prescribe the minimum effective dose, and treat the resident for as short a time as possible.

Antidepressant Drugs

Depression is common among nursing home residents, and is underdiagnosed and undertreated. It may cause a wide variety of disturbing behaviors, including agitation, aggression, wandering, sleep disorders, crying, and loss of interest in usual activities.

Simple assessment tools, such as the Geriatric Depression Scale, may be of little use in a resident with dementia or a resident who is unable to communicate. For such residents, anecdotal evidence may be more useful than results of formal assessment instruments. Every member of a resident's care team, as well as family members, should be asked whether they have noticed any symptoms of depression. Where diagnosis is difficult, physicians sometimes decide to treat the resident for depression and to watch for signs of improvement. Treating depression is frequently of value even if the patient has significant dementia.

In selecting an antidepressant, it is important to match the drug to the resident. No one drug—not even fluoxetine (Prozac)—is appropriate for every depressed patient. Stimulating antidepressants should generally not be prescribed for residents who are anxious. Sedating antidepressants should be used only as a last resort in residents who already sleep much of the time. At the Hebrew Home of Greater Washington, staff often prescribe nortriptyline (Pamelor) for residents with uncomplicated depression who have no heart problems that would contraindicate its use; trazodone (Deseryl) at bedtime for residents with major sleep disturbances; and methylphenidate (Ritalin) for residents with vegetative symptoms or residents in whom a rapid response is needed. Psychiatric consultation is strongly advised for residents whose cases are not straightforward.

Sedatives and Hypnotics

Many older adults have difficulty sleeping, and many enter nursing homes after years of taking sedatives and hypnotics. Despite overwhelming evidence that these drugs lose their effectiveness after only a few weeks, and that they are often responsible for increased falling, many residents and their families resist having these drugs discontinued. To reduce the use of sedatives and hypnotics, staff need to educate families and residents about the dangers associated with sleeping medications. If the resident agrees to do so, he or she should be switched to one of the shorter-acting hypnotics, such as temazepam, and the frequency of the dose should be reduced gradually over a period of a few weeks until the resident is free of the drug.

Despite the knowledge that the use of barbiturates as sedatives is inappropriate, some older adults have been taking these drugs for many years. Due to the physiologic addiction these dangerous substances cause, a very slow dose reduction is necessary.

No sleeping pill is totally safe for older adults. Antihistamines, such as diphenhydramine (Benadryl), produce significant side effects, including sedation and urinary retention, and they, too, increase the likelihood of falling. The most appropriate approach in treating sleeping problems is to try to determine why the resident is sleeping poorly. If he or she experiences physical discomfort, a bedtime dose of an analgesic may be helpful. The need to get up frequently at night to urinate is another common cause of disturbed sleep. Reducing fluid intake in the evening and adjusting the timing of the resident's medication may help reduce the need to urinate.

Finding the Right Dosage

For older adults, the range within which a psychotropic drug produces desirable effects without significant side effects—the "therapeutic window"—is very narrow. Blood level readings for psychoactive drugs are of limited use in older adults. Hence, any adjustments in a resident's drug dosage should be based on clinical observations.

Finding an effective dosage of a drug that does not cause marked lethargy seems to be a particular problem with residents with vascular dementia. Many of these residents present the greatest behavior management challenges. For them, repeated psychiatric consultation is appropriate.

Prescribing Psychotropic Drugs on an "As Needed" Basis

Ordering psychotropic drugs on an "as needed" (prn) basis should be avoided, except under special circumstances, described in this section. Prn use may lead to underuse or overuse of the drug, depending on how comfortable the nursing staff is in dealing with the resident's behavior. The resident's well-being is adversely affected by the swings in behavior caused by intermittent drug use. At the Hebrew Home of Greater Washington, staff prefer to start patients on a regular, low dose of an appropriate drug. The dosage is increased gradually every few days until the resident experiences the desired effect. Once the resident calms down, the physician may decrease the dosage so that the resident does not become lethargic. To adjust the dosage in this way, the physician must be in frequent contact with the nursing staff who see the resident daily.

A prn order may be appropriate for a resident receiving a regular dose of a psychotropic drug who sometimes needs additional treatment. However, the order must be specific enough for a staff member who does not know the resident to decide whether to give the prn dose. An order for "Haldol 0.5 mg im or po prn" is not adequate. The order should specify the target behavior requiring treatment as well as the dosage limit. A more appropriate order might be; "Haldol 0.5 mg prn for aggressive behavior (attempting to hit others). May be repeated q4h if needed for maximum of 3 doses in 24 hours. Give im if resident will not take po." If the resident's symptoms frequently require prn doses, the regular dose of antipsychotic should be increased. If the prn dose is not needed for 30–45 days, it should be discontinued, since a change in behavior after that period would justify re-evaluating the resident to determine the cause.

Prescribing Psychotropic Drugs for Residents Whose Behavior Disturbs Other Residents

Sometimes highly agitated residents behave in ways that are deeply upsetting to other residents. Newly admitted residents with moderate dementia, for example, often behave in ways that affect the well-being of others. At the Hebrew Home of Greater Washington, in cases in which the new resident has no medical problems that need urgent attention, the dosage of psychotropic drugs administered is increased rapidly until the new resident is calm. The dosage is then gradually reduced, allowing the resident to adjust slowly to the new surroundings.

SELECTING TREATMENT GOALS AND EVALUATING EFFECTIVENESS

For all psychiatric diagnoses, the attending physician and the rest of the staff must cooperate in carrying out three processes:

1. Establishing the goals of the resident's treatment
2. Monitoring the effectiveness of the treatment and adjusting the resident's drug dosage
3. Observing the resident for side effects and drug interactions

Establishing Treatment Goals

Just as the care team would establish a blood pressure goal in treating a resident's blood pressure, it must establish behavioral treatment goals in treating behavioral symptoms. To do so, the caregivers must be able to measure the resident's symptoms. Because most behavioral symptoms are episodic, it is easiest to quantify them in terms of how often they occur. For example, how many times a day does the resident become combative? How often does the resident refuse treatment? How often does the resident wander off the unit? In order to determine whether treatment has been effective, the care team must determine a baseline of a resident's behavior over a period of time (e.g., 2–7 days). Once the baseline behavior is recorded, the effects of therapy can be evaluated.

Monitoring the Effectiveness of Treatment and Adjusting the Resident's Drug Dosage

The assessment of behavioral symptoms must be based on multiple observations. This tracking of behavior over a period of several days is shown in the following case study:

Mr. Kent, an 86-year-old widower, has lived at Pinehurst Manor for 7 months. He entered the facility after his fractured hip was repaired. Although his recovery was good, he had significant cognitive impairment and could no longer function in the community. In the past several weeks, Mr. Kent began striking his tablemates during meals. He became verbally abusive with staff when they did not respond immediately to his needs. Medical and psychiatric assessment found no cause for this change in behavior, other than dementia. His score on the Folstein Mini-Mental State Examination was 12. The psychiatric consultant suggested that he take 0.5 mg of haloperidol a day and that his behavior be monitored.

Monitoring by staff on all shifts showed that Mr. Kent acts out about 15 times a week. Since Mr. Kent's behavior seems to be triggered by external events, it may not be possible to eradicate his outbursts completely without making him lethargic. The initial treatment goal was to reduce the number of episodes to no more than one a day by having staff eliminate the external events that seem to elicit his aggressive behavior (i.e., having to wait for his food). To this end, they moved his seat in the dining room closer to the serving area and tried to make sure that his food was served as quickly as possible. Little change occurred the first week, and Mr. Kent's dose of haloperidol was increased to 0.5 mg three times a day. Although he seemed drowsy for a few days, he returned to his usual level of alertness, and the number of aggressive episodes fell to three to five a week.

Even though the psychiatric consultant started Mr. Kent on an antipsychotic drug, the care team implemented environmental and behavioral interventions.

Monitoring for Side Effects and Drug Interactions

All psychotropic drugs can produce major side effects, including addiction, sedation, anxiety, urinary retention, hypotension (extremely low blood pressure), and tardive dyskinesia (involuntary movements). When psychotropics are administered to a resident who is already taking one or more other potent medications, the combination may be disastrous. For example, administering a sedating drug to a resident who is constantly sleepy or lethargic could cause such a resident to be unable to feed him- or herself or to recognize when he or she needed to urinate. Prescribing a psychotropic drug with hypotensive side effects to a resident with low blood pressure could cause such a resident to fall, to become confused, or to faint. Certain combinations of drugs can even result in death. It is thus crucial that the physician carefully consider what medications the resident is already using before he or she prescribes a new psychotropic agent. Since many residents with difficult behavior also suffer from other major medical conditions and may thus be taking many potent medications, the physician may need to consult with a professional knowledgeable about the psychopharmacology of drugs in older adults.

One very common serious side effect of psychotropic medication is tardive dyskinesia, which causes involuntary movements of the lips or jaw, as well as other parts of the body. Tardive dyskinesia is common in older adults, and has been tied to the use of antipsychotic and antidepressant drugs. It may occur immediately with the first dose of a drug, even at very low dosages, as well as after prolonged use or high dosage. Although residents are generally not disturbed by the involuntary movements associated with tardive dyskinesia, families often find these movements distressing. To minimize the frequency and severity of these effects, all residents who are to receive drugs that may cause tardive dyskinesia should be assessed for involuntary movements before they start treatment and while they are on treatment. Assessment should be done at least every 6 months while the drug is being used. A number of assessment instruments such as the Abnormal Involuntary Movement Scale (AIMS) have been proposed, but none has been generally accepted as of this date.

DETERMINING WHEN TO DISCONTINUE TREATMENT

The most common abuse of psychotropic drugs occurs when drugs continue to be administered after the resident no longer requires them. Because the OBRA '87 regulations apply not only to new residents but also to residents who were taking psychotropic medications before the regulations went into effect, long-term care facilities have been trying to reduce dosages or eliminate the use of psychotropic drugs in all residents, in order to comply with the federal regulations. Unfortunately, there are no data to guide the caregiver in determining how long a resident should continue to take a psychotropic drug, and the reduction in dosage or discontinuation of psychotropic drugs may not be appropriate for all residents.

For example, the medical record of one resident gave no indication as to why that resident had been placed on an antipsychotic drug. Because no current evidence indicated that the drug was needed, the dosage was tapered and the drug eventually discontinued. After a few months, the resident began to display grossly psychotic behavior. Despite the reinstitution of the medication, the symptoms could not be controlled and the resident was admitted to a psychiatric hospital. Only after much probing did the family recall that the resident had been diagnosed as psychotic several years earlier and had responded well to antipsychotic medication. To prevent such a situation from occurring, caregivers who are unable to find documentation regarding the reason a drug was initially prescribed should question the family and others who may recall the circumstances prompting the initial administration of the drug. If the caregivers are unable to discover why the drug was started, the dosage should be lowered gradually, with the guidance of a consulting psychiatrist.

Caregivers should keep in mind that the resident's condition changes over time, and that problem behaviors may appear and disappear without any intervention. If the resident continues to exhibit the problematic behavioral symptoms, the drug should probably be continued. If, however, the problem behavior occurs only infrequently, the physician may decide to reduce the dosage and monitor the resident's behavior. If the reduction in the dosage is not associated with an increase in problem behavior, the dosage may be reduced further until it is discontinued altogether or until a level is found at which the problem reappears.

DOCUMENTING THE USE OF PSYCHOTROPIC DRUGS

Documentation of the use of psychotropic drugs is crucial, but often woefully neglected in long-term care facilities. As Garrard and colleagues note (1991), even when psychotropic drugs appear to have been used appropriately, documentation supporting their use is often inadequate. The importance of documenting drug use for all residents cannot be overstated. For every resident receiving psychotropic medication, the following information must be recorded:

1. The resident's behavior problem
2. The diagnosis underlying the problem
3. The treatment objective
4. The treatment selected
5. The effectiveness of the treatment
6. Evidence of side effects
7. Changes in treatment
8. The need for continued treatment
9. The next date the treatment will be evaluated

Such documentation complies with the intent of the 1987 OBRA regulations, and allows the resident's care to be monitored. In order to ensure that proper documentation is done for all residents at the Hebrew Home of Greater Washington, a form (shown in Figure 10.1) was created. After several months, use of the form became unnecessary because the medical staff became familiar with the documentation required and preferred to include it with their regular progress notes.

In addition to the federally required case-by-case review of all psychotropic drug use by the consulting pharmacist, the Hebrew Home of Greater Washington utilizes facility-wide tabulation of all psychotropic drug use in order to monitor trends and changes. (A sample is shown in Table 10.3.) The purpose of compiling such data is

---

PSYCHOTROPIC DRUG REVIEW

Resident's name: _____

Current drugs, dose, and frequency: _____

Change in target behavior symptoms: _____

Side effects noted: _____

Recommendations (check one or more as appropriate):

( ) a. Change dose of _____ to _____
        because of _____

( ) b. Discontinue current medication because _____

( ) c. Start new medication _____ at dose _____

( ) d. No change in medication is appropriate because of
        _____

Date: _____ Reviewer(s): _____

Figure 10.1. Sample form for recording psychotropic drug use by residents.

Table 10.3. Sample facility-wide tabulation of psychotropic drug use

		Number of residents on			
Unit	Number of residents	Antipsychotics	Anxiolytics	Antidepressants	Sedative hypnotics
A	38	8	5	11	5
B	37	7	2	3	4
C	38	4	8	6	3
D	38	9	5	7	6
E	36	14	5	4	4
Total	187	42	25	31	22
Percent of residents on drugs in class		22.5	13.4	16.6	11.8

not to compare one unit with another, but to look at trends over time. This tool is helpful to medical staff, and can become part of the facility's quality assurance program.

CONCLUSION

The 1987 OBRA regulations, as well as the principles of good medical care, require that caregivers think carefully about their patient care practices. A caregiver's response to difficult behavior must not be simply to administer a sedating drug. Instead, the initial response must be to try to find the cause of the behavior. Only after making a presumptive diagnosis can the caregiver consider what would be the most appropriate treatment. In many cases, behavior management, examined in Chapter 14, can represent an alternative to drug treatment.

Where treatment with psychotropic drugs is necessary, they should be used carefully and residents should be monitored and assessed for evidence that the drug is effective or evidence that the drug causes unacceptable side effects and should be discontinued. Meticulous documentation, indicating a description and diagnosis of the resident's problem, the treatment objective, the drug and dosage prescribed, evaluation of the effectiveness of the drug, evidence of side effects and therapeutic effect, and any changes in the dosage or the medication itself must be kept on all residents given psychotropic drugs.

Before treating a resident with a psychotropic drug, the caregiver must take the following steps:

1. Treatment goals should be identified in terms of behaviors that need to change.

2. At the time the drug is ordered, a preliminary decision should be made about when to evaluate the effectiveness of the treatment. Evaluations may need to take place every few days (or even more often) initially.

3. The drug should be titrated to the level that will achieve the desired effect or to the level of tolerance in terms of side effects.

4. If an effective dosage cannot be found without causing the resident to experience significant side effects, the treatment should be changed.

5. If the treatment is effective, the resident should be monitored at least every 60–90 days to determine whether he or she still requires treatment.

6. If the resident's condition is stable, the physician may consider tapering the drug and discontinuing it if the resident no longer needs it.

7. Monitoring for signs of tardive dyskinesia should be done when a resident is started on an antipsychotic or an antidepressant drug and at least every 6 months while they continue to receive it.

REFERENCES

Beers, M., Avorn, J., Soumerai, S., Everitt, D.E., Sherman, D.S., & Salem, S. (1988). Psychoactive medication use in intermediate-care facility residents. *Journal of the American Medical Association, 260*(20), 3016–3020.

Garrard, J., Makris, L., Dunham, T., Heston, L.L., Cooper, S., Ratner, E.R., Zelterman, D., & Kane, R.L. (1991). Evaluation of neuroleptic drug use by nursing home elderly under proposed Medicare and Medicaid regulations. *Journal of the American Medical Association, 265*(4), 463–467.

Health Care Financing Administration. (1989). Medicare and Medicaid; requirements for long term care facilities. *Federal Register, 54*, 5316–5336.

Health Care Financing Administration. (April, 1992). Interpretive guidelines. *State Operations Manual*, Transmittal 250.

Jenike, M.A. (1989). *Geriatric psychiatry and psychopharmacology: A clinical approach.* Chicago: Year Book Publishers.

Johnson, J.F., & DiBona, J.R. (1990). A concurrent quality assurance review of psychotropic prescribing in elderly patients: Process and outcome measures. *Journal of Geriatric Drug Therapy, 4*(4), 43–80.

Lantz, M., Louis, A., Lowenstein, G., & Kennedy, G. (1990). A longitudinal study of psychotropic prescriptions in a teaching nursing home. *American Journal of Psychiatry, 147*(12), 1637–1639.

Sloane, P.D., Mathew, L.J., Scarborough, M., Desai, J.R., Koch, G.G., & Tangen, C. (1991). Physical and pharmacologic restraint of nursing home patients with dementia. *Journal of the American Medical Association, 265*(10), 1278–1282.

Part IV

Clinical Issues in Restraint Use

Chapter 11

Understanding Falling, Wandering, Agitation, and Immobility

Vivian J. Koroknay, Patricia Carter,
Jeanne R. Samter, and Renee Clermont

Physical and chemical restraints are usually used in response to falling, wandering, and agitation. This chapter examines each of the major reasons for restraining older adults and examines the effects of prolonged immobility on the musculoskeletal, cardiovascular, respiratory, gastrointestinal, renal, and integumentary (skin) systems of older people. Finally, it examines the behavioral effects of restraints in older adults.

FALLING

Fall-related injuries are a serious problem for older adults. Among older adults living independently, approximately one-third of those over 65 and half of those over 80 fall each year (Tinetti, 1990). When disease accompanies the aging process, as is often the case with nursing home residents, falls are even more likely to occur. Among residents of long-term care facilities, a fall rate of two falls per resident per year has been reported (Baker & Harvey, 1985). Both the chance of falling and the chance of sustaining serious injury from a fall rise as people age (Brummel-Smith, 1989; Stone & Chenitz, 1991; Waller, 1985).

For many years, long-term care facilities restrained residents who had fallen or who appeared likely to fall. This practice was believed to prevent residents from hurting themselves. Recent research has demonstrated that restraints may actually cause residents to fall, and that they may produce some of the injuries sustained during falls (Powell, Mitchell-Pedersen, Fingerote, & Edmond, 1989; Tinetti, 1987).

Factors that predispose an older adult to fall may be divided into two categories, intrinsic and extrinsic (Stone & Chenitz, 1991). Intrinsic factors include normal aging changes, the use of certain medications, and the presence of disease or illness. Extrinsic factors are environmental conditions, such as poor lighting or slippery floors. Falls among older adults are often caused by intrinsic factors that impede the person's ability to cope with extrinsic (environmental) factors (Waller, 1985).

Intrinsic Factors

Many intrinsic factors are associated with falls in older adults. Age-related changes in posture and balance, gait, and vision that predispose older people to falls are examined here. Other intrinsic factors associated with falls are identified in Table 11.1.

Posture and Balance   The term *posture* refers to the alignment of body parts in relation to one another (Kauffman, 1990). One of the most noticeable orthopedic changes associated with age is the change in posture. In normal posture, the ear, shoulder, hip, knee, and ankle align in a straight line. In older adults, however, the head tends to lean forward, the shoulders may be rounded, and the upper back may have a slight curvature, or kyphosis. Postural abnormalities increase when there is a decline in strength and flexibility. Changes in spinal alignment can affect balance, thus increasing the risk of falling (Kauffman, 1990).

Postural sway, which is characterized by movement of the upper body when the feet are stationary, is associated with the aging process. This phenomenon causes postural instability, and is associated with falls (Brummel-Smith, 1990; Rhymes & Jaeger, 1988). The body's ability to maintain its coordination in a standing position and to react to prevent itself from falling depends on the ability of the musculoskeletal system, neurosensory system, and visual system to work together. Postural sway occurs when these systems lose their ability to coordinate and maintain the body's balance.

Postural reflexes maintain postural stability by responding to disturbances in balance when a person is standing or walking. In older people, these reflexes are diminished and the motor response is slower. Therefore, older people are less able to make postural corrections and are more likely to fall when there is a change in balance (Rhymes & Jaeger, 1988). Inactivity may also account for this slower reaction time in response to balance disturbances (Riffle, 1982).

Table 11.1. Intrinsic factors associated with falls in older adults

History of falls
Changes in balance and gait
Postural hypotension
Visual impairment
Cognitive impairment
Diminished memory or recall ability
Weakness/deconditioning
Underlying illness
Infection
Pain
Podiatric conditions
Medications
Incontinence/fear of incontinence
Problem behavior (wandering, agitation, socially inappropriate or disruptive behavior)
Immobility (causing weakness and decreased flexibility)

Muscle weakness, which is common among older people, primarily affects the legs. Because the muscles that work against gravity are most affected, standing up can become difficult. This leg weakness is associated with falls among residents of long-term care facilities (Tinetti, 1987).

Decreased strength and response in the muscles of the ankles are also common in older people. This may be a particular problem since they are less capable of readjusting to changes in the body's center of gravity when there is a loss of balance (Stone & Chenitz, 1991).

Gait The normal gait pattern consists of two phases, the stance phase and the swing phase. Changes in the gait pattern of older adults occur in both phases, and include the following:

- shortened steps
- decreased foot pick up
- decreased arm swing and body rotation
- decreased velocity
- irregular steps

In the stance phase, which accounts for 60% of the normal walking cycle, both feet are on the ground (Spector, 1991). Most problems become apparent in the stance phase, because it is the weight-bearing phase of gait. Joints and muscles undergo the greatest stress in this phase (Mensch & Ellis, 1986).

In the swing phase, the muscles of the hip must hold the pelvis level while the body weight is on one leg as the other leg swings by to take the next step. Both flexibility and strength at the hip, knee, and ankle joints are needed to swing the leg in this phase (Mensch & Ellis, 1986). During this phase of gait, the muscles of the ankle, knee, and hip must work together to clear the foot from the ground. For many older people, this motion is difficult. This decreased step height may result in tripping falls.

Another consequence of aging is decline in muscle coordination, which decreases the ability of the pelvis to shift toward the weight-bearing leg during walking. Because the pelvis is still shifted onto the non–weight-bearing leg, it may swing forward too low, making it difficult for the person to lift the leg over an obstacle and causing the person to fall(Stone & Chenitz, 1991).

By the time a person reaches his or her 60s or 70s, there is a noticeable decrease in muscle strength (Gioiella & Bevil, 1985). This diminished muscle strength, along with decreased joint flexibility, causes older people to feel insecure in the one-legged stance position of the swing phase. The response is a slower gait and a shortened step height.

An important change that occurs as people age is the reduction in the normal speed of walking, which falls by 50%–60%. This drop in walking speed below the efficient level means that more energy is consumed by walking, resulting in greater fatigue. Slower walking is responsible for greater fatigue (Spector, 1991), which in turn causes falls to occur more often (Brummel-Smith, 1990). Many of the older adult's gait patterns reflect the body's attempt to minimize the amount of energy expended in walking (Spector, 1991).

Older people walk with decreased arm swing and body rotation because there is less automatic motion in the gait. In normal gait, there is a natural forward sway of the body. In the swing phase, there is a forward sway as the heel contacts the ground and the body moves over it. In the stance phase, there is a forward sway as the foot is again moved over the ground at the end of the cycle. In older adults, forward sway is typically reduced because of increased tightness in the hip muscles and decreased flexibility in the hip joint.

Vision   All older people experience changes in vision as a result of the normal aging process, with approximately 90% of people over 65 needing corrective lenses (Stone & Chenitz, 1991). Aging brings a decline in visual acuity, peripheral vision, depth perception, night vision, tolerance for glare, and ability to focus on objects at different distances (Kline & Schieber, 1985; Stone & Chenitz, 1991). In the aging eye, pupil size becomes smaller, and less light reaches the retina. This reduces the pupil's ability to dilate and constrict in response to changes in light (Ebersole & Hess, 1985). Consequently, moving from a well-lit hall into a darkened room is particularly difficult for older people.

The loss of visual acuity that accompanies aging means that approximately one third of people over 80 have vision of 20/50 or less. This means that these people can identify at 20 feet or less what a person with normal vision can identify at 50 feet or less. The ability to focus on objects at a distance and judging distance also declines. The effect of this visual change can be seen when an older person misses a step on a curb and falls. In addition, the decline in peripheral vision that accompanies aging may cause the older person to trip over objects at the edge of the visual field.

Coupled with the normal visual changes that accompany aging is the relatively high incidence of diseases that further impair vision in older people. A study of 112 long-term care facility residents found that 83.9% of those studied had cataracts, 28.6% had age-related disease of the macula, 1.8% had a degenerative disease of the retina, and 3.6% had glaucoma (Horowitz, 1988).

Vision is important to maintaining stability both while walking and while standing still (Brummel-Smith, 1989). A visual deficit can compound an older adult's gait disability (Overstall, 1985) and can make him or her more likely to fall (Riffle, 1982; Snipes, 1983; Stone & Chenitz, 1991). Changes in visual field also affect a person's perception of where his or her body is in relation to other structures in the environment. This, too, makes falls more likely (Tinetti & Speechley, 1989).

Adequate lighting is essential to the older person's safety. Because the diameter of the pupil is decreased, the amount of light that reaches the retina of an older person is only one-third of that reaching the retina of a younger person (Kline & Schieber, 1985). A 60-year old requires twice as much light to see as does a 20-year old. As a result, walking becomes dangerous, especially in poorly lit areas (Ebersole & Hess, 1985).

Too much light can also be detrimental to an older person's vision, because of the increased sensitivity to glare. The large windows and highly polished floors so often found in long-term care facilities can distort the older person's vision and make obstacles difficult to see.

Because of the age-related changes in vision that affect older adults, vision assessment for every resident is an important part of a fall prevention program. Staff members should receive education about the importance of corrective lenses in preventing falls. The resident should not be considered fully dressed if he or she wears glasses but does not have them on. Factors in the facility's physical environment, too, can compound the effects of diminished vision and make falls more likely, as the next section explains.

Extrinsic Factors

It is important that staff understand how both intrinsic and extrinsic factors affect the safety of older people. Extrinsic factors include various aspects of the physical environment that may precipitate falls. Such factors include clutter in the halls, glare in common areas, and inadequate lighting in residents' rooms. At least 50% of older adults' falls result from such environmental factors (Ebersole & Hess, 1985). Facilities must address these issues if they are to lessen the number of falls for their residents. Some of the extrinsic factors of special concern in long-term care facilities are listed in Table 11.2.

Living in an environment that is not designed with the older adult's safety needs in mind can diminish a resident's confidence. As the person comes to feel less secure, either because of a fear of falling or because of a previous fall, he or she may become more sedentary. Eventually, such inactivity may lead to a loss of function and an increase in the person's dependence on others, neither of which is in keeping with a restorative care approach.

Lighting Proper lighting is important for people with normal vision as well as those with impaired vision. In many facilities, halls and room lighting are at opposite extremes—halls are often too bright and rooms are dark and shadowy. Older people have difficulty adjusting to such stark changes in light. Moving from a bright area to a darker environment takes additional time for the eye to adapt, and may cause an older person to experience a temporary loss in vision. Very bright light can cast heavy shadows and create dark areas that can cause the resident to fall due to perceptual deficits in the visual field. Residents should be able to control the amount of light in their rooms by having different types and levels of lighting available.

Keeping bedrooms and bathrooms completely dark at night is a dangerous practice for residents who must get up during the night to use the bathroom. Low voltage night lights may reflect shadows and these images may be misinterpreted, possibly causing a resident to

Table 11.2. Extrinsic (environmental) causes of falls in older adults in long-term and acute-care settings

Inadequate lighting
Shiny, slippery floors
Long hallways
Clutter in halls
Spills on the floor
Bathrooms with inadequate grab rails
Slippery bathroom floors
Furniture not designed for older people (e.g., beds, chairs, or toilets that are too high or too low, tables or beds whose wheels do not lock)
Inappropriate footwear
Clothing that is too big
Equipment in resident/patient areas

fall when going to the bathroom. Leaving a higher voltage light on at night may reduce the resident's confusion and in some cases may actually promote sleep.

Furniture   In both the home and the facility, most falls occur in the bedroom and the bathroom (Rhymes & Jaeger, 1988). Falls are most likely to occur in these areas because people spend most of their time there and because of the hazards associated with these rooms.

Furniture should provide stability and support, and should be arranged so that walking areas remain uncluttered. A study by Overstall (1985) found that nursing home residents fall most often while moving from bed to chair or while sitting on or rising from the toilet. Particular attention should be made to making these areas safe. Beds and chairs that are too high and toilets that are too low can cause residents to lose their balance. To ensure safety, beds and chairs should be no higher than 18 inches from the floor (Tideiksaar, 1990). Staff should assess the need for bedrails carefully, since many falls occur when residents attempt to climb over them. Bed wheels must lock securely so that the bed does not move when the resident is getting into or out of bed. Items kept next to the bed, such as call lights, television controls, mobility aids, and toileting equipment, must be accessible, so that residents do not fall trying to reach them (Stone & Chenitz, 1991). Chairs should have firm support cushions to provide a stable base for safe seating, armrests that extend to the front of the chair for safe exiting, and a stable support base to prevent tipping. Equipment such as overbed tables and carts with wheels may be hazardous to the resident who holds on to these devices when walking. Staff should make sure that residents do not lean on this equipment.

Clothing Clothing can affect the older person's safety. Since clothing that is loose fitting and too long often causes falls, well-fitting clothing is crucial for older people. Poorly fitting shoes can impede mobility and cause a person to fall. Shoes should fit properly and provide firm support without being too cumbersome or heavy. Rubber soles and low-heeled shoes tend to reduce the number of falls caused by slipping, although ribbed rubber-soled shoes may catch on carpeting.

WANDERING

Wandering is a very serious problem in nursing homes, and one that is of grave concern to administrators and clinicians. Prevention of wandering has traditionally been a major reason for restraining residents. Caregivers' knowledge of the reasons that underlie wandering has expanded considerably since Burnside addressed this problem in *Psychosocial Nursing Care of the Aged* (1980), and this understanding should enable caregivers to seek alternatives to restraints in dealing with wandering behavior.

Wandering is defined as the tendency "to move about, either in a seemingly aimless or disoriented fashion, or in pursuit of an indefinable or untouchable goal" (Snyder, Rupprecht, Pyrek, Breknus, & Moss, 1978, p. 272). Residents may wander from a room or activity, from the floor of the facility, or from the facility itself.

Like other nonverbal behaviors, wandering is a form of communication that can be understood in terms of its components. Milke (1989) studied behaviors that preceded residents' attempts to leave the floor of their facility and found a high correlation between trespassing (i.e., entering a barred area) and leaving. The fact that certain behaviors tend to precede wandering should provide staff with a way of monitoring residents' activities. For example, after observing a resident's wandering behavior, staff may recognize that prior to leaving the floor the resident enters the staff lounge. Rather than use restraints, staff may simply keep an eye on the resident, watching in particular for movement toward the lounge. Once the resident enters the lounge staff can divert his attention with an activity.

Wandering by New Residents

Some of the more severe forms of exit seeking have been observed to occur in residents who have been recently admitted. New residents tend to feel unsettled and suffer from a tremendous sense of loss. These residents tend to get up frequently in the night, sometimes pacing in their rooms, sometimes rummaging through the belongings of other residents. Their wandering has a searching quality that may express the sense of loss they feel.

Residents who exhibit unsettled behavior upon admission have traditionally been treated with neuroleptics as the first line of therapy. Initially, such drugs may be effective in reducing the resident's movements, since they cause drowsiness. Eventually, however, such medications tend to aggravate their agitation. They are thus not consistent with a restorative approach to care.

New residents at the Hebrew Home of Greater Washington have responded positively to a treatment regime that addresses the stress they experience upon moving to the facility. Interventions that are appropriate for preventing wandering are presented in Table 11.3. Such interventions require the commitment of all staff members in helping new residents adjust to their surroundings. When staff work together to help new residents adjust, this settling-in period is often easier. Sleep patterns are stabilized and the residents look more alert and are better able to participate in group activities. Residents who receive such treatment are also much less likely to wander. A facility that seeks to reduce the use of restraints should thus implement some sort of regime to reduce the stress of relocation for new residents.

The ambivalence and anxiety that families feel about placing a

Table 11.3. Interventions for preventing wandering

Request that all staff members support residents in every way they can, especially if they appear to be wandering because of relocation stress.

Help residents find their places on the unit.

Befriend residents.

Make eye contact with residents.

Walk arm in arm with residents.

Have a volunteer accompany residents outdoors.

Encourage residents to follow any favorite routines from the past.

Promote the use of rituals.

Encourage families to visit frequently.

Agree with residents' statements rather than challenge or refute them.

Observe the nature of residents' wandering by staying alert to patterns.

Try to determine the meaning of the behavior from the residents' viewpoint.

Request a psychiatric consultation to assess residents for depression.

Transfer residents to units where they may wander safely.

family member in a nursing home often contribute to the new resident's feelings of uncertainty and may cause the resident to wander. Staff should work with families to help them overcome these feelings and communicate a sense of security to the newly admitted resident.

Wandering by Other Residents

Exit-seeking is not limited to new residents. Even stable residents who have been in the facility for years may attempt to leave. For residents who are cognitively intact, this behavior may reflect their frustration or depression. In impaired residents, exiting may herald a decline in cognitive function.

Traditionally, caregivers dealt with exit-seeking behavior by trying to eliminate it, even if doing so meant putting the resident in the most restrictive environment as a first-line intervention. A restorative care approach attempts to understand the exit seeking from the point of view of the resident. Staff can then implement strategies that will assist residents to remain as functional as possible without having to move to more restrictive units. The following case studies demonstrate a restorative care approach in dealing with exit seeking.

> Martha Williams, an 82-year old resident of Wayland Nursing Home, began making attempts to leave the facility after reporting that the facility's food was inedible. Rather than devise ways of preventing Mrs. Williams from wandering, the staff first held a care conference to try to understand the factors that precipitated Mrs. Williams' behavior. They determined that Mrs. Williams' declining physical status had caused her to worry about becoming totally incapacitated, and that her wandering may have represented her attempts to establish her independence.
>
> The team devised an increased support plan that included more attention from all staff members and weekly one-on-one therapy with the social worker. The dietitian worked with the Mrs. Williams to vary the menu to suit her tastes. Staff also encouraged the family to visit more often during this crucial period. Within the month, Mrs. Williams stopped trying to leave.

In some cases, a more restrictive environment is the appropriate intervention. However, it is important that other measures be tried first, as the following case study demonstrates:

> Eighty-seven year old Isaac Wolfson began leaving the unit daily. He was often found in the basement near the boiler room. Sometimes he wandered as far as the parking lot.

The resident's only son objected to having his father moved to a more secure unit because of the present unit's proximity to the facility's synagogue. Mr. Wolfson, a Jewish immigrant from Poland who spoke no English, had been deeply religious all his life, and had attended daily prayer sessions since entering the facility. His son believed that the ritual of daily services provided comfort to his father. Staff agreed that Mr. Wolfson seemed to benefit from his religious rituals despite his severe dementia. Until his most recent decline, the services had helped to provide structure to Mr. Wolfson's day.

For several months, Mr. Wolfson had appeared highly disoriented. He became agitated in the closed environment of his unit. A Yiddish-speaking psychiatrist evaluated Mr. Wolfson's mental status and conducted a care conference with staff. He encouraged staff members to allow Mr. Wolfson to remain on the unit, where he had lived for several years. After the conference, the staff redoubled their efforts to make nonverbal contact with Mr. Wolfson and to support him however possible. The son hired a companion for his father for a couple of hours every day.

For a time, these interventions were successful: for 6 weeks, Mr. Wolfson made no attempt to leave. After 6 weeks, however, Mr. Wolfson once again began to wander. The staff requested that he be moved to a locked unit for his own safety.

The issue of a residents' safety is an important one, which cannot be overlooked. However, it is important to handle residents' attempts to leave as sensitively as possible and in a manner that addresses the need underlying the behavior. The nature of caregivers' thinking about wandering affects their selection of interventions. Since the goal in restorative care is to maximize an individual's self-care capacity, caregivers should seek out and employ measures that promote residents' physical and mental capacity for adjustment with the least amount of restrictions.

AGITATION

Agitation is common in nursing home residents, and needs to be dealt with immediately, both to ensure the comfort of agitated residents and to prevent them from becoming aggressive. Traditionally, interventions consisted of the application of physical restraints and/or the medication of the resident with neuroleptics. Since the implementation of the OBRA '87 regulations, however, facilities have been looking for alternative ways to manage agitation.

Although agitation is common in nursing homes, it is poorly understood by direct care staff, whose jobs are often limited to completion of specific tasks. Nursing assistants who are occupied with bathing, ambulating, and toileting residents often have too little time to try to understand the reasons underlying a resident's agitation.

Agitation is not a disease but a symptom, a human response to a physical or emotional problem. It may manifest itself in the form of wandering, restlessness, irritability, repetitive motor activity, sleep disturbances, or aggression. Although it is common in older people, it is not an inherent part of the aging process.

Agitation may be associated with physical or psychological illnesses that require treatment. Often, residents with severe dementia will reveal their depression through agitated behaviors. A facility that wants to help its agitated residents rather than merely restrain them must understand the source of the agitation. A thorough assessment of the resident is crucial.

The Classification of Agitation

Agitation may be classified by the effect it has on the resident and on others in the environment. Zimmer, Watson, and Treat (1984) describe four categories of agitation:

1. Harmful to self
2. Harmful to others
3. Disturbing to others
4. Nonharmful or nondisturbing but troublesome to staff

Different types of agitated behaviors seem to appear together (Cohen-Mansfield, 1988). For example, residents who bite often kick and hit as well. Residents who are cognitively intact manifest agitation differently from those who have impairments. Residents with dementia may dress inappropriately or disrobe. Cognitively intact residents may hoard or hide things, express negative attitudes, or complain excessively. Recognizing the different ways in which different types of residents react can help staff members who care for agitated residents predict these behaviors and plan accordingly.

Sources of Agitation

Physiological Sources Physiological causes of agitation include cardiac diseases, congestive heart failure, infections, drug toxicity, drug withdrawal, and drug interactions. Constipation and dehydration severe enough to produce electrolyte imbalance and fatigue as a result of sleep deprivation may also cause agitation in older adults.

Older people who are cognitively impaired and cannot express pain verbally may express their feelings nonverbally via agitation, as seen in the following case:

Wilma Brown, an 80-year-old resident, was seen thrashing about in her wheelchair. She was restrained to prevent her from falling. Observing her behavior, a staff member reported it to the physician, who ordered a psychiatric evaluation. When the psychiatrist visited the facility, he found Mrs. Brown to be demented but unagitated. Given the odd pattern of her behavior, the charge nurse inferred that Mrs. Brown's thrashing reflected physical discomfort. Further assessment revealed that Mrs. Brown was taking Procardia. Suspecting that the resident was experiencing an increase in chest pain, the nurse asked the physician to examine Mrs. Brown. After examining her, he increased the dosage of Procardia. One month later, the resident was doing well and no further episodes of agitation occurred.

Psychological Sources The most prominent psychological factor precipitating agitation is relocation stress. This phenomenon is common after a resident moves to a long-term care facility or moves from one unit in the facility to another. Any change in the resident's lifestyle or family system can create psychological stress.

Each resident responds differently to the stress of relocation, and different approaches and different modes of treatment are appropriate for these reactions. If the resident is experiencing an adjustment reaction, staff should implement supportive measures to ease this transition. Activities such as taking a bath at a certain time of day, following a walking routine, or celebrating certain holidays or other events in a special way can help stabilize a resident who is suffering from stress associated with transition. Other steps for dealing with agitated residents are shown in Table 11.4. If depression, inactivity, or agitation persist, psychiatric intervention may be appropriate.

Environmental Sources Many factors contribute to a chaotic living environment for residents of long-term care facilities. Residents with dementia may be unable to screen out stimulation from the environment. Unlike cognitively intact residents, they cannot use internal mechanisms, such as daydreaming, to avoid the distractions presented by the environment. As a result, they may find even mildly stimulating environments overly stimulating. The routine activities that take place daily in the facility may also contribute to the residents' agitation. Noise from loudspeakers, the constant ringing of telephones, and the coming and going of staff on the unit floor are constant features in long-term care facilities that may agitate some residents. Other events, such as visits by families and friends, fire drills, or the death or hospitalization of other residents, can also cause agitation.

When the environment appears to be overly stimulating, staff

Table 11.4.   Intervention for preventing and dealing with agitation

Teach staff how to recognize warning signs, particularly an increase in motor activity (e.g., pacing, humming, crying out).

Educate staff about environmental precipitants of agitation.

Assess the resident for constipation, fatigue, pain, and infection.

Make as few demands on residents as possible when they appear agitated.

Listen to the residents' feelings rather than try to cheer them up.

Provide a quiet place for agitated residents, away from stimulation.

Nurture, reassure, and comfort agitated residents.

Allow residents as much control over their daily lives as possible (e.g., offer them bounded choices, such as "Would you like to sit here and be quiet, or go to your room?").

Learn about residents' interests before they become agitated, and reward them with time to pursue these activities if they cooperate with caregivers.

Plot the time and frequency of the residents' episodes of agitation and try to correlate these episodes with what is happening in the environment.

Evaluate residents' responses to different interventions, noting what works and what doesn't.

Ask family members to visit more often when residents seem to be having a particularly difficult time.

---

should first determine whether anything can be done to modify the environment to make it more sedate. Staff should be instructed to keep their voices as low as possible, to avoid shouting across halls, and to modify their body movements so that they are slow and purposeful rather than quick and confusing.

When it is not possible to alter the environment, it may be helpful to remove the resident to a quiet alcove for a brief interlude. Sometimes establishing an afternoon rest period—either a nap or quiet time for a specific interval each day—can increase a resident's ability to cope with the stimulation of unit routines, such as shift changes.

Medication   Medication may provoke agitation. Since aging retards metabolism, drugs are eliminated more slowly and possibly absorbed less thoroughly in older people than they are in younger people. Drugs may accumulate in the body, resulting in toxicity that is sometimes manifested as delirium. Although psychotropic drugs have been effective in controlling mental illness, they may precipitate or prolong agitation. Caregivers need to watch residents who are on psychotropic medications carefully for signs of drug-induced agitation.

Withdrawal from medications, especially those of the benzodiazepine group, is also a common cause of agitation. When a resident is to be removed from a drug, the dosage must be tapered gradually, to prevent hallucinations, paranoia, or other forms of agitation.

EFFECTS OF PROLONGED IMMOBILITY

Prolonged immobility resulting from restraint use can cause many adverse effects in older people. When older adults are immobilized by restraints, all of their major body systems are likely to become impaired. Some of these changes are irreversible and may subsequently affect the person's health. Because older adults' physical reserves are limited due to the normal changes that accompany aging, and because they often suffer from chronic illnesses, they are especially susceptible to the negative effects that follow immobilization by restraints.

As a result of prolonged immobility, older adults can experience serious biochemical, physiological, and psychological effects, as shown in the following sections (Harper & Lyles, 1988; Miller, 1975).

Effect on the Musculoskeletal System

A progressive decline in bone density is a normal consequence of aging (Gioiella & Bevil, 1985). In addition to this normal decline, older people who are confined to a bed or chair lose some of their weight-bearing capacity, causing further bone dissolution (Miller, 1975). As a result, older adults who are restrained are much more likely to develop osteoporosis. Possible consequences of osteoporosis include fractures of the hip, spine, and extremities, all of which further limit mobility (Mobily & Kelley, 1991).

Another consequence of immobility is nitrogen loss, which indicates loss of muscle. When a person is immobilized, muscle strength diminishes by approximately 5% per day, with the leg muscles losing strength about twice as fast as the arm muscles. Muscle atrophy occurs from the 2nd through the 10th day of immobility. Muscle wasting occurs faster when the muscles are in a shortened position. This means that older people who are confined to beds or chairs are at a particular risk, since they tend to flex their arms and legs when at rest (Gioiella & Bevil, 1985; Harper & Lyles, 1988).

Generalized muscle weakness is a normal change that accompanies aging. The result is a decrease in muscle strength that becomes noticeable in a person's 60s and 70s. This loss of strength places older adults at particular risk of developing severe muscle weakness if they are confined to bed- or chairrest. Research has found that weakness of the legs is a predictor of falls in long-term care facility residents (Tinetti, 1987). Because the muscles that work against gravity are most affected, standing up becomes the most difficult movement. In time, the ability to walk, to balance, and to turn around becomes severely impaired (Browse, 1965; Mobily & Kelley, 1991), predisposing people with weakened muscles to falls. Hence, the immobility that results from restraint use increases the risk of falling.

Other changes in the muscoskeletal system that occur with bedrest can further increase an older person's risk of falling. Disordered motor functioning of the voluntary muscle groups has been noted in immobilized residents who attempt to stand (Miller, 1975). Immobility also compromises the body's ability to maintain coordination when standing upright. These changes are characterized by an increase in postural sway (Harper & Lyles, 1988). Like weakness of the legs, postural sway is also a predictor of falls and has been associated with prolonged bedrest as well as with aging in general (Tinetti, 1990).

Joints are severely affected by immobility. Older adults can develop 90° contractures of the knees and hips from sitting all day in a chair and lying in bed at night without straightening their legs (Gioiella & Bevil, 1985). Because the joints no longer bear weight, changes occur in the tissue in and around the joints that are very similar to the changes associated with arthritis (Harper & Lyles, 1988). Within as little as a week after a person has been confined to bed, changes in the cartilage of the joints can occur that make the joints less flexible. If not corrected, permanent loss of mobility can occur in the joint (Harper & Lyles, 1988).

Effect on the Cardiovascular System

Older adults who are immobilized by restraints may also suffer from changes that occur in the cardiovascular system. Many of these changes are closely associated with inactivity. Both cardiac output and the cardiovascular response to exercise diminish as a natural result of aging and as a consequence of bedrest (Harper & Lyles, 1988; Timiras, 1988). In a person who has been immobile for more than 2 weeks, the decline in cardiac output will be twice as great as in a person who has not been confined to bed (Harper & Lyles, 1988).

Another consequence of extended bed- or chairrest is a decrease in blood pressure when the person stands up. The longer a person stays in bed, the more frequently he or she will experience orthostatic hypotension and dizziness upon standing up (Browse, 1965). The prevalence of this complication also increases with age (Cunha,

1987). This makes older adults who have been immobile for long periods more likely to fall as a result of changing their body position, and may cause them to fear walking (Hoenig & Rubenstein, 1991).

Effect on the Respiratory System

Changes in the respiratory system place older adults at risk of developing respiratory complications as a result of decreased mobility. Normal changes in the aging body that compromise the functioning of the lungs include increased rigidity of the rib cage, kyphosis, and osteoporosis. These changes tend to make the chest wall less flexible (Gioiella & Bevil, 1985).

By the age of 70, changes in the alveoli and structural changes in the lung tissue result in a marked decrease in the vital capacity of the lungs (Bennison & Hogstel, 1986). Impaired ventilation and decreased blood supply to the lungs are likely consequences of the decrease in the amount of lung surface area available for gas exchange and the loss of elasticity in the lung tissue of older adults (Timiras, 1988). Coupled with immobility, these anatomical changes increase the risk that some portions of the older person's lungs will be unable to expand to receive air and an atelectasis (collapse of the lung) will occur. Hence, the older client is at high risk of developing hypostatic pneumonia and possibly dying as a result of bed- or chairrest (Bennison & Hogstel, 1986; Harper & Lyles, 1988; Mobily & Kelley, 1991).

Effect on the Gastrointestinal System

The prolonged immobility that results from restraint use may cause older adults to suffer from appetite loss, weight loss, and dehydration (Evans & Strumpf, 1989; Miller, 1975). Appetite loss may be caused by hypercalcemia, a condition that occurs when the circulating blood contains an abnormally high concentration of calcium compounds. This condition occurs when the bones demineralize as a result of prolonged immobility. Another condition associated with loss of appetite may be a prolonged negative nitrogen balance, which occurs as a result of muscle wasting and begins after a person has been immobile for 5–6 days(Miller, 1975). These factors, together with the already diminished appetite common to many inactive older adults, increase the risk of malnutrition as a result of being immobilized (Behnke, 1986).

Water balance in older adults is compromised as a result of the aging process. Age-related changes that predispose the person to dehydration include a decrease in total body water content, an altered sense of thirst, a decrease in kidney function that makes the kidneys unable to respond to changes in the person's physical health, and a decrease in the effectiveness of the body's antidiuretic hormone (Kositzke, 1990). Because of the net loss of total body water that occurs with bedrest, older adults are at increased risk for dehydration (Harper & Lyles, 1988; Kostizke, 1990). Immobility, underlying illnesses, and multiple drug use further increase the risk of dehydration in older patients or residents.

In hospitalized older adults whose activity is limited, food takes longer to move through the gastrointestinal tract than in non-hospitalized, active older adults (Harper & Lyles, 1988). The muscle atrophy and loss of muscle tone that occur in a patient or resident who is immobilized, malnourished, and weakened affect the efficiency of the muscles that are involved in elimination (McCarthy, 1967). In addition, when residents' or patients' usual elimination patterns are disrupted, or when they must suppress the urge to eliminate because they are unable to get to the toilet, constipation and/or incontinence of stool often result (McCarthy, 1967). Hence, being restrained not only compromises the physiological mechanism of elimination, but also prevents the individual from being able to meet such basic self-care needs as going to the toilet.

Effect on the Renal System

Like gastrointestinal function, urinary function is strongly affected when older adults are restrained. The renal and excretory systems function optimally when the body is erect. When the body is supine or immobilized by restraint use, patients or residents are likely to suffer from a number of urinary tract complications (Mobily & Kelley, 1991). These include urinary incontinence, urinary retention, formation of kidney stones, and urinary tract infections (Browse, 1965; Harper & Lyles, 1988).

A number of age-related changes in the excretory system of older people may make them more likely to be incontinent when they are prevented from using the toilet by use of a restraint. In older adults, bladder capacity diminishes to about half that of younger adults. The diminished ability of the kidneys to concentrate urine also causes older people to need to urinate frequently, and to experience the need to urinate at night (Gioiella & Bevil, 1985). Older adults tend to have uninhibited contractions of the detruser muscle of the bladder, which may cause urinary urgency. Urgency and frequency may eventually cause urinary incontinence in a person who is restrained, since the restraint limits the person's ability to go to the toilet as quickly or as often as needed, or to summon help to go to the toilet. In fact, new-onset incontinence has been found to result

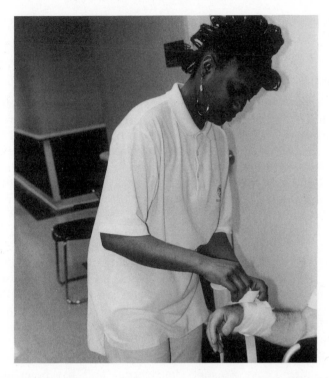

Protective padding around the wrist helps prevent damage to the delicate skin of the older person who is restrained. (Photograph courtesy of the Hebrew Home of Greater Washington. Used by permission.)

directly from restraint use (Lofgren, MacPherson, Granieri, Myllenbeck, & Srrafka, 1989; Warshaw et al., 1982).

Effect on the Integumentary (Skin) System

The effects of immobility on older adults' skin are well known. Restraints and the immobility that results from them increase the risk of developing pressure ulcers. When a person is lying down, the weight of the body is redistributed from the feet, which are well-adapted to bearing the body's weight, to other areas of the body that are less able to bear such weight (Browse, 1965).

Aging skin also increases a person's likelihood of developing pressure ulcers. As the body ages, the blood supply to the skin diminishes, there is less subcutaneous tissue, and changes occur in the epidermal and dermal layers that cause the skin to become more fragile (Timiras, 1988). This means that the skin of older people is less resistant to the effects of immobility than that of younger people, and that older people are at greater risk for developing pressure ulcers when they are immobilized.

BEHAVIORAL EFFECTS OF RESTRAINTS

The feelings of emotional desolation and the disorganized behaviors that often occur when a resident is restrained may result from the perceptual and behavioral responses to being immobilized (Evans & Strumpf, 1989). Misik (1981) has noted that patients and residents often react with feelings of panic, embarrassment, and hostility when confined by restraints, and that they often feel that they are being punished. Agitation may also increase when restraints are used (Werner, Cohen-Mansfield, Braun, & Marx, 1989). In a study of residents in a long-term care facility who were restrained for at least 4 weeks, Miller (1975) noted that a number of behavior and mood changes occurred. These included an increase in depression, fear, and panic, and a worsening of preexisting paranoia and symptoms of organic brain syndrome. The residents studied also exhibited regressive behavior, becoming more withdrawn socially and more apathetic. Often, they stayed in the fetal position when in bed, and some became stuporous.

Restricting a resident's freedom of movement by using restraints may cause sensory deprivation and psychosis (Covert, Rodrigues, & Solomon, 1977; Harper & Lyles, 1988). Because older adults' hearing and vision are often impaired, sensory deprivation can occur very easily. Many cognitive changes result from sensory deprivation, including, but not limited to, confusion, disorientation, and a general slowing of intellectual activity, as manifested by difficulty in concentration, thinking coherently, and solving problems (Gioiella & Bevil, 1985). These symptoms may be labeled incorrectly as "senility," thus providing further justification for restraint use.

REFERENCES

Baker, S., & Harvey, A. (1985). Fall injuries in the elderly. *Clinics in Geriatric Medicine, 1*(3), 501–508.

Behnke, M. (1986). Anorexia. In V.K. Carrieri, A.M. Lindsey, & C.M. West (Eds.), *Pathophysiological phenomenon in nursing* (pp. 99–121). Philadelphia: W.B. Saunders.

Bennison, B., & Hogstel, M. (1986). Aging and movement therapy: Essential interventions for the immobile elderly. *Journal of Gerontological Nursing, 12*(12), 8–16.

Browse, N.L. (1965). *The physiology and pathology of bedrest.* Springfield, IL: Charles C Thomas Publisher.

Brummel-Smith, K. (1989). Falls in the aged. *Primary Care, 16*(2), 377–391.
Brummel-Smith, K. (1990). Falls and instablity in the older person. In
    B. Kemp, K. Brummel-Smith, & J. Ramdell (Eds.), *Geriatric rehabilitation*
    (pp. 193–208). Boston: Little, Brown.
Burnside, I.M. (1980). *Psychological nursing care of the aged.* New York:
    McGraw Hill.
Cohen-Mansfield, J. (1988). Agitated behaviors and cognitive functioning in
    nursing home residents: Preliminary results. *Clinical Gerontologist 7*(3/4),
    11–22.
Covert, A., Rodrigues, T., & Solomon, K. (1977). The use of mechanical and
    chemical restraints in nursing homes. *Journal of the American Geriatrics
    Society, 25*(2), 85–89.
Cunha, U. (1987). Management of orthostatic hypotension in the elderly. *Ger-
    iatrics, 42*(9), 61–65.
Ebersole, P., & Hess, P. (1985). *Toward healthy aging: Human needs and nurs-
    ing response* (2nd ed.). St. Louis: C.V. Mosby.
Evans, L., & Strumpf, N. (1989). Tying down the elderly: A review of the liter-
    ature on physical restraints. *Journal of the American Geriatrics Society, 37,*
    65–74.
Gioiella, E., & Bevil, C. (1985). *Nursing care of the aging client.* Norwalk, CT:
    Appleton-Century-Crofts.
Harper, C., & Lyles, Y. (1988). Physiology and complications of bedrest. *Jour-
    nal of the American Geriatrics Society, 36*(11), 1047–1054.
Hiatt, L. (1986). Effective trends in interior design. *Provider, 12,* 28–30.
Hoenig, H., & Rubenstein, L. (1991). Hospital-associated deconditioning and
    dysfunction. *Journal of the American Geriatrics Society, 39*(2), 220–222.
Horowitz, A. (1988). The prevalence and consequences of visual impairments
    among nursing home residents. *Monograph of the Lighthouse, Inc.* New
    York, NY.
Kauffman, T. (1990). Impact of aging-related muscoloskeletal and pos-
    tural changes in falls. In C. Lewis (Ed.), *Topics in geriatric rehabilitation:
    Balance and falls* (Vol. 5, No. 2, pp. 34–44). Rockville, MD: Aspen
    Publications.
Kline, D.W., & Schieber, F. (1985). Vision and aging. In J.E. Birren & K.W.
    Sehaie (Eds.), *Handbook of the psychology of aging* (pp. 296–331). New
    York: VanNostrand Reinhold.
Kositzke, J. (1990). A question of balance: Dehydration in the elderly. *Journal
    of Gerontological Nursing, 16*(5), 4–11.
Lofgren, R., MacPherson, D., Granieri, R., Myllenbeck, S., & Srrafka, J.
    (1989). Mechanical restraints on the medical wards: Are protective devices
    safe? *American Journal of Public Health, 79*(6), 735–738.
McCarthy, J. (1967). The hazards of immobility: Effects on motor function.
    American Journal of Nursing, 67, 4.
Mensch, G., & Ellis, P. (1986). Introduction to lower extremity amputations.
    In G. Mensch & P. Ellis (Eds.), *Physical therapy management of lower ex-
    tremity amputations* (pp. 1–20). Rockville, MD: Aspen Publishers.
Miller, M. (1975). Iatrogenic and nurisgenic effects of prolonged immobility
    of the ill aged. *Journal of the American Geriatrics Society, 23*(8), 360–369.
Milke, D.L. (1989). *Wandering in dementia: Behavioral observations.* Unpub-
    lished manuscript. University of Alberta. Edmonton, Alberta, Canada.
Misik, I. (1981). About using restraints with restraint. *Nursing '81, 11*(8), 50–
    55.

Mobily, P.R., & Kelley, L.S. (1991). Iatrogenesis in the elderly: Factors of immobility. *Journal of Gerontological Nursing, 17*(9), 5–11.

Overstall, P.W. (1985). Falls. In M. Pathy (Ed.), *Principles and practice of geriatric medicine* (pp. 701–709). New York: John Wiley & Sons.

Powell, C., Mitchell-Pedersen, L., Fingerote, E., & Edmond, L. (1989). Freedom from restraint: Consequences of reducing physical restraints in the management of the elderly. *Canadian Medical Association Journal, 141*, 561–564.

Rhymes, J., & Jaeger, J. (1988). Falls: Prevention and management in the institutional setting. *Clinics in Geriatric Medicine, 4*(3), 613–622.

Riffle, K. (1982). Falls: Kinds, causes, and prevention. *Geriatric Nursing,* May–June, 165–169.

Snipes, G. (1983). Analysis and prevention of falls. *Geriatric Consultant,* May–June, 22–25.

Snyder, L.H., Rupprecht, P., Pyrek, J., Breknus, S., & Moss, T. (1978). Wandering. *The Gerontologist, 18,* 272–280.

Spector, M. (1991). Gait and gait training in the elderly. In J. Glickstein (Ed.), *Focus on geriatric care and rehabilitation* (Vol. 4, No. 10, pp. 1–8). Rockville, MD: Aspen Publications.

Stevens, G.L., Baldwin, B.A., Eigelsbach, L.M., & Friedman, S.D. (1991). *Stress and behavioral management in long-term care: A motivation training manual.* Baltimore: National Health Publishing.

Stone, J., & Chenitz, W. (1991). The problem of falls. In W. Chenitz, J. Stone, & S. Salisbury (Eds.), *Clinical gerontological nursing* (pp. 291–306). Philadelphia: W.B. Saunders.

Tideiksaar, R. (1990). Environment adaptations to preserve balance and prevent falls. In M. Woollacott (Ed.), *Topics in geriatric rehabilitation, 5*(2), 78–85. Rockville, MD: Aspen Publications.

Timiras, P. (1988). *Physical basis of aging and geriatrics.* New York: MacMillan.

Tinetti, M. (1987). Factors associated with serious injury during falls by ambulatory nursing home residents. *Journal of the American Geriatrics Society, 35*(7), 644–648.

Tinetti, M. (1990). Falls. In C. Cassel, D. Reisenberg, L. Sorenson, & J. Walsh (Eds.), *Geriatric medicine* (2nd ed., pp. 529–534). New York: Springer-Verlag.

Tinetti, M., & Speechley, M. (1989). Prevention of falls among the elderly. *New England Journal of Medicine, 320*(16), 1055–1059.

Waller, P. (1985). Preventing injury to the elderly. In H.T. Phillips & S.A. Gaylord (Eds.), *Aging and public health* (pp. 103–146). New York: Springer Publishing.

Warshaw, G., Moore, J., Friedman, W., Currie, C., Kennie, D., Kane, W., & Mears, P. (1982). Functional disability in the hospitalized elderly. *Journal of the American Medical Association, 248,* 847–850.

Werner, P., Cohen-Mansfield, J., Braun, J., & Marx, M. (1989). Physical restraint and agitation in nursing home residents. *Journal of the American Geriatrics Society, 37,* 1122–1126.

Zimmer, J.G., Watson, N., & Treat, A. (1984). Behavioral problems among patients in skilled nursing facilities. *American Journal of Public Health, 74*(10), 1118–1120.

Chapter 12

Activities as Alternatives to Restraints

Barbara D. Fleischmann and Barbara E. Van Hala

When federal nursing home reforms took effect on October 1, 1990, residents' rights became the watch word. The mandate of the Omnibus Budget Reconciliation Act of 1987 to provide the least restrictive environment possible for nursing home residents created new challenges for activities professionals. As a result of this legislation, therapeutic recreation and activities departments are now being called upon to play greater roles in creating or implementing activities specifically designed to be consistent with the restraint-free philosophy.

Activities, once viewed by other health care professions as little more than diversionary games, are now being recognized as therapeutic interventions, systematically planned to deal with behavior problems that once would have elicited the use of chemical and physical restraints. An agitated resident may be calmed for periods of time by listening to soft music; a wandering resident can be distracted from exit seeking by participating in an exercise or dance session. While activities are not the only interventions that can be used as alternatives to restraints, they are important adjuncts to other interventions and are critical in a total restorative care approach.

Although little has been written about the types of activities that may be used in place of chemical or physical restraints, advocates of restraint-free environments encourage the use of activities as restraint alternatives (Blakeslee, 1989). The key to using activities as therapeutic alternatives to restraints is successfully to match appropriate activities with residents based on their individualized assessments, their plans of care, and their abilities and needs. By engaging residents in appropriate structured activities programs, the therapeutic recreation and activities staff attempts to minimize or eliminate the behavior previously necessitating restraints.

The therapeutic recreation and activities department must address multiple problematic behaviors when developing programs in a restraint-free environment. Some behaviors are:

- Wandering and pacing
- Restlessness and agitation
- Anger and physical and verbal aggression
- Disorientation due to a change in environment
- Frustration, depression, and withdrawal due to limiting physical conditions and abilities

This chapter examines a variety of activities that can be used to meet residents' physical, emotional, cognitive, and social needs. Activities can be used to:

- Channel excess energy into physical activities.
- Reduce stress and relieve anxieties with relaxation techniques.
- Stimulate mental functioning through cognitive or educational opportunities.
- Raise the spirits through creative expressions.
- Redirect behaviors into appropriate social means.

All may be considered alternatives to restraints if used with appropriate residents and incorporated into their individualized plans of care. The last section of this chapter looks at the role of activities in implementing a restorative care philosophy in the long-term care setting.

GOALS OF THERAPEUTIC RECREATION AND ACTIVITIES

A therapeutic recreation and activities program should include activities that 1) promote physical, cognitive, social, and emotional health; 2) enhance self-respect by providing opportunities for self-expression, personal responsibility, and choice; and 3) provide stimulation or solace to residents who do not generally benefit from the traditional therapeutic recreation and activities program. In the past, the goal of the activities programs—to optimize resident participation and experiences—had been difficult to achieve because of the use of restraints, which often prohibited a resident from fully participating in an activity. A resident who preferred activities that required walking, for example, was forced into the role of passive observer as long as he or she was physically restrained. Chemical restraints also impeded a resident's ability to engage fully in meaningful activities.

A therapeutic recreation and activities program that reinforces the quality of life and restorative care philosophy, encourages restraint reduction, and supports a restraint-free environment will incorporate the following goals:

- Respect each resident and motivate each person toward participation according to background, interest, and capabilities;
- maintain, encourage, and/or restore social and recreational outlets for all residents, whether ambulatory or nonambulatory;
- improve social interaction among residents, staff, and family members;
- assist in the adjustment process that each resident faces upon admission and throughout his/her stay at the facility;
- design individualized programs for those residents who prefer solitary leisure or who are unable to function in a group setting;
- provide alternatives for residents who due to deteriorating health, have experienced functional losses in cognitive, physical, social, and emotional areas;
- modify programs to provide success-oriented activities in the least restrictive environment; and create and initiate new activity programs on a continuous basis in relation to the changing population of the facility. (Fleischmann & Van Hala, 1982, p. 6)

These goals have traditionally been included in therapeutic recreation and activity programming. The new approach of a restraint-free environment necessitates the inclusion of an additional goal:

Modify and create activities to aid in reducing stress and agitation, anxiety, wandering, and other behaviors that were previously controlled with restraints.

Success-oriented activities used in therapeutic recreation and activities programs and the corresponding program goals and safety considerations promoting a restraint-free environment are examined in this chapter. Specific programs of physical activities, relaxation and stress reduction activities, cognitive and educational activities, creative expression activities, and social activities are described. Success-oriented programs are simple and easy to institute. They take advantage of retained skills, nurture the resident, and provide meaningful experiences that build self-esteem. All of the techniques and programs examined can be easily adapted for use by any member of the interdisciplinary team.

PHYSICAL ACTIVITIES

Physical activities are essential to a restorative care approach. Exercises, range of motion, rhythmic movements, gross motor games, and walking offer residents the opportunity to move, stretch, flex, and extend. The objectives of physical activities programs are shown in Table 12.1.

Safety considerations are important when planning and implementing programs requiring physical exertion by the residents. Strenuous physical activity by adults with chronic disabilities can be dangerous. Even mild to moderate exercise by someone with compromised cardiac function or someone who has been immobile for a prolonged period of time can result in injury or harm. Particular attention needs to be given to assessing the capabilities of the resident and planning exercises or physical activities that are within his or her tolerance level. Table 12.2 provides guidelines for ensuring that physical activities remain safe.

Physical activities should also be modified depending on environmental factors. For example, activity sessions should be shortened and made less demanding when the weather is very hot or humid or air quality is poor. General guidelines for conducting physical activities are listed in Table 12.3.

Exercise Programs

Exercise is valuable at every age. In older adults, exercise can help to improve strength, flexibility, balance, and coordination. Because of chronic disabling conditions and minimal opportunities for physical activity, nursing home residents frequently live sedentary lives.

Table 12.1. Objectives of physical activities

Increase energy capacity.
Channel excess energy into appropriate activity.
Maintain and/or increase physical stamina and endurance.
Increase muscular strength.
Tone muscles and improve posture.
Improve circulation, especially to the limbs.
Stimulate and aid in digestion.
Increase mental acuity.
Reduce boredom and mental fatigue.
Improve sleep patterns.
Decrease wandering, agitation, and stress.

Table 12.2. Guidelines for ensuring that physical activities remain safe for all participants

Obtain a physician's approval.

Observe residents for signs of overexertion, shortness of breath, overexcitement, or verbal or nonverbal signs of pain. If such signs are observed, stop exercise and notify the nurse in charge.

Monitor heart rate during strenuous exercises.

Shorten the time of the session, and/or lessen the intensity of the activity when the weather is very hot or humid, or air quality is poor.

During the activity, place all residents in view of the leader.

Check all equipment regularly for needed maintenance.

Make sure equipment is properly adapted to suit the needs of the residents.

Scale down the weight of manipulated objects (e.g., use a nerf or beach ball in place of a basketball).

When tossing objects, aim for the lower body, away from the face.

Planning and implementing a regular exercise program within the facility will promote general fitness and increased mobility.

Exercise programs for older adults, particularly frail nursing home residents, must be approached with a degree of caution. The resident's current level of fitness should first be assessed in a thorough history and physical exam, and any exercise program should be initiated only with a physician's approval.

Procedures should be established to determine each resident's exercise tolerance. Monitoring heart rate prior to exercise and periodically through the session is one means of identifying exercise intolerance. To find the maximum heart rate, the activity leader should subtract the resident's age from the number 220. The target

Table 12.3. Guidelines for conducting physical activities

Minimize distracting noise or movement in the surrounding environment.

Space residents at least one arm's length apart to allow room for movement of arms.

Use simple words of instruction with an enthusiastic and an energetic tone.

Use residents' names frequently to encourage and maintain interest.

Demonstrate body movements in an exaggerated fashion when explaining range of motion activities or games such as modified volleyball or basketball.

Arrange chairs and wheelchairs in a circular formation to encourage social interaction.

Instruct residents to hold hands palms up to receive thrown balls.

Use music to vary the mood.

heart rate is 60%-80% of this number. Thus, to find the target heart rate during exercise for a healthy 70-year-old, the activity leader would subtract 70 from 220 and find 60%–80% of that number. The lower figure, 90, represents the lower bound of the desired range. The higher figure, 120, represents the upper bound of the desired range. Strenuous exercise resulting in significant increases in the heart rate is not recommended, unless stress testing is done prior to participating in an exercise program. The leader of the exercise group should also observe for other signs of exercise intolerance. Such signs include dizziness, angina, nausea, confusion, marked shortness of breath, and fainting (Barry, 1986). Exercise should be terminated if a resident exhibits any of these signs.

Exercise programs for older adults should be conducted three to five times per week, and should involve low-intensity activities that involve the large muscle groups (Barry, 1986). A warm-up period of exercise, allowing time for the body to prepare to work out, is important. This 5- to 10-minute period of slow movement allows the blood to circulate to all extremities before participants engage in full range of motion movements. Warm-up exercises prepare the circulatory system for exertion and prevent musculoskeletal injuries (Barry, 1986; Glickstein, 1991).

After warm-up, the exercise activities may increase in difficulty. Exercises should be aimed at developing flexibility, strength, or endurance in the various muscle groups. Flexibility exercises include easy stretching and developmental stretching. Stretching exercises help maintain joint mobility and flexibility. The resident should be encouraged to use full range of movement.

Developing muscular strength and endurance through exercises is achieved through dynamic contraction, in which the muscle is allowed to shorten. Contraction exercises include pulling rubber exercise tubing, exercising with light weights, and performing calisthenics (Weiss, 1988).

Another component of fitness is the aerobic endurance phase of exercises. Aerobic activities involve the use of large muscle groups, which are exercised continuously in a rhythmic manner for a sustained period of time. Walking or riding a bicycle are examples of aerobic activities. Aerobics exercises can also be done while sitting. Aerobic activity elevates the heart rate into the training range. A study of 53 sedentary older women living in the community demonstrated significant improvement in cardiorespiratory endurance, strength, body agility, flexibility, and balance for the subjects participating in a 12 week low-impact aerobic dance program (Hopkins, Murrah, Hoeger, & Rhodes, 1990). Body fat was also reduced. For

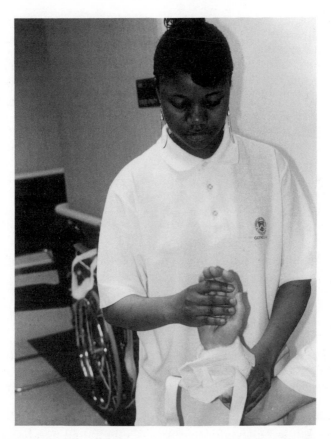

To prevent loss of function, staff need to perform range of motion exercises with patients or residents who are restrained. (Photograph courtesy of the Hebrew Home of Greater Washington. Used by permission.)

residents who are able, commercially produced exercise videos, such as Richard Simmons' "Silver Foxes Low Impact Aerobics," can be used. Residents should continuously move the upper and lower extremities to achieve cardiovascular fitness. The actual time for the more challenging exercise phase will vary depending on the exercise tolerance level of the individual, but normally can be scheduled to last 12–20 minutes.

Equally as important as a warm-up period is a cool-down period. Cooling down is accomplished by lessening the intensity and duration of the exercise, and including more frequent rest periods. Cool-down activities permit the gradual redistribution of blood flow, and allow the dissipation of body heat (Weiss, 1988). Water and juices should be available and offered to participants at the end of the session or during the session as necessary to replace fluid loss through perspiration (Glickstein, 1991).

Exercise programs must be modified to meet the needs of the residents involved. For more ambulatory and agile residents, exercise can be performed from a standing position. For other residents, exercises can be conducted from a sitting position in a chair or wheelchair. Examples of specific exercises for immobile older adults can be found in Benison and Hogstel's article on aging and movement therapy (1986).

The leader may use music or add props to alter the intensity or form of the activity. Incorporating music or choreographing specific routines makes the exercise period more enjoyable and is a good way of retaining residents' interest. Adding an assortment of props to the exercise routines provides variety and sparks residents to put more energy or effort into their movements. Table 12.4 lists some of the props that can be used during exercise sessions.

Gross Motor Games and Activities

Any activity that allows the body to move, provides practice in hand —eye coordination, or provides amusement for the residents can be a gross motor game activity. Gross motor games can be included in an exercise session or be scheduled as a separate activity for the residents' enjoyment. Several gross motor games are listed in Table 12.5.

Modified Sports

Sports such as volleyball, tennis, basketball, and baseball can be modified for frail older adults by adapting equipment and/or changing the rules of the game. For instance, a basketball hoop can be lowered to a more accessible height of about 4—5 feet from the ground. Light-weight tennis rackets can be made by stretching a pair of pantyhose over a wire hanger bent into an oblong shape with handle, and a balloon can be used for the tennis ball. The rules of the game can be modified to make the game easier, and to allow more residents to participate.

Organized Walking Clubs

Walking programs are gaining popularity in nursing homes and have been used in some hospitals as well as efforts increase to combat immobility. Such programs can help to strengthen muscles, improve ambulatory status, and foster independence (Koroknay, Werner, Cohen-Mansfield, & Braun, 1991; Norman & Gibbs, 1991; Orr & DeProspero, 1991). The therapeutic recreation and activity depart-

Table 12.4. Props that can be used by older adults during physical activities

Props	Use
Batons and canes	Batons and canes can be used for stretching and twisting.
Flags	Used along with march music, flags provide an incentive to move. Waving a flag or saluting a flag involve movements of the upper extremities.
Rhythm sticks	Rhythm sticks can be used during exercises by clacking them together, twirling them, or moving them from one hand to another. Drums can be beaten to promote a greater sense of rhythm.
Shakers or maracas	Handmade or purchased shakers or maracas can be used to promote a greater sense of rhythm during exercise.
Streamers	Handheld ribbons or ribbons attached to dowel rods can be used to encourage rhythmic gymnastic movements.
Stretch elastics	Residents use elastics to provide resistance while working the muscles of their arms and legs. Stretch elastics can be made by sewing the ends together of a 2-foot long by 1-inch wide piece of elastic.

ment can provide structured walking programs and staff supervision for groups of walkers. Residents also enjoy walking with staff, with volunteers, with their families, and with each other either throughout the nursing home or outdoors. Many nursing homes have walking clubs, with awards for miles walked.

RELAXATION AND STRESS REDUCTION ACTIVITIES

Older adults admitted to long-term care facilities experience considerable stress. Not only must they acclimate to the stresses of institutionalized living, they must also cope with losses resulting from disease, disabilities, and separation. Facility staff must be sensitive to the changing physical, mental, and emotional needs of residents, and be creative in providing them opportunities to vent emotion, release tension, and redirect energy. Relaxation and stress reduction activities can thus be valuable alternatives to restraints. Program objectives for relaxation and stress reduction activities are shown in Table 12.6.

Relaxation techniques and agitation reduction activities can take many forms. Some examples are breathing exercises, visual

Table 12.5. Gross motor games that can be used as physical activities

Game	Description and purpose
Ball toss and catch	Residents can sit or stand in a circle while the leader stands in the middle and tosses a soft or large ball to each participant. The resident returns the ball by tossing it to the group leader.
Darts	Darts with suction cups on the end can be thrown at a target.
Hokey pokey	The popular children's game of "put your right hand in, put your right hand out" can be used with older adults as an enjoyable method of moving large muscles of the arms and legs.
Hot potato	Residents sit in a circle and pass a ball to the next person. The game can be varied by changing the pace of the game.
Kick the ball	Residents kick or push a ball as an enjoyable way of promoting lower extremity movement.
Target toss	Residents try to toss a ball, bean bag, or other object into a target, such as a box or waste paper basket.
Velcro mitts and ball	Baseball mitts with Velcro make catching a sponge ball easy. Residents with limited strength or range of motion may benefit from using.

imagery, dough kneading, yoga, and repetitive calming tasks. In these types of activities relaxation is the main goal. Guidelines for conducting relaxation and stress reduction activities are shown in Table 12.7.

Breathing Exercises

Shallow breathing, used in everyday life, can increase stress and tension. Deep breathing, or diaphragmatic breathing, promotes relaxation. Progressive muscle relaxation exercise done in conjunction with deep breathing can enhance the relaxing effect. These exercises use the process of tightening and releasing major muscle groups, thus varying the sensations of tension and relaxation. Since improper breathing techniques can result in light headedness and dizziness, caution and keen observation is essential during such exercises.

Easy Listening

Background music can help reduce agitation in some residents. Residents who benefit from background music may show signs of relax-

Table 12.6. Objectives of relaxation and stress reduction activities

Foster stress-free participation.
Reduce agitation, anxieties, and other problematic behavior.
Allow residents opportunity to fantasize.
Promote feelings of self-worth and sense of well-being.
Provide outlet for venting emotions.
Help residents recognize stress factors.
Instruct residents in self-management of own stressors.
Validate group experiences.
Allow opportunities to release built-up tension.
Channel negative behavior into constructive avenues.

ation, such as decreased movement or drooping eyes. However, other residents may become agitated by the music, and may show increased restlessness, muscle tension, or vocalization. Since background music affects residents in different ways, caregivers must observe residents to determine the effect the music has on them. Music that results in increased agitation should be eliminated immediately. The same music may be introduced at another time so that its effect can be reassessed.

Like younger people, residents have different tastes in music. To accommodate the range of musical preferences, the facility should encourage the use of tape players with earphones.

Housekeeping Brigade

Involvement in routine activities performed in the past, such as housekeeping tasks, often reduces anxiety in older adults. Residents with early- to mid-level dementia sometimes enjoy pushing a broom

Table 12.7. Guidelines for conducting relaxation and stress reduction activities

Set the mood and be an active participant.
Be aware of distracting noises in the environment.
Conduct the session in a calm, quiet room.
Close the door to shut out outside distractions.
Modulate your voice to promote a calming and soothing environment.
Allow residents to vent anxieties, fears, and other feelings.
Validate experiences of the resident.
Encourage residents to share their own coping methods.
Select only calming background music or use no music.

or using a sponge to wipe surfaces. A resident's behavior may indicate a preference for this type of activity. A resident who walks endlessly, touching and smoothing surfaces, may enjoy using a dust cloth. Residents' preferences for these activities can be identified by discussing their earlier habits with their families. Family involvement is critical when planning an activity of this sort, as families must understand that such activities represent therapeutic relaxation activities, and are not meant to replace staff responsibilities.

Tension Busters

Many activities and tasks can be used to lessen agitation, reduce tension, and redirect energy. Tension busting activities may include calming and soothing tasks, such as folding towels, counting rosary beads, and rolling yarn. Structured activities to release aggression and excess energy, such as kneading dough or crushing aluminum cans for recycling, can also serve this purpose.

Pets

Pets can have a positive and therapeutic effect on nursing home residents (Weisberg & Pack, 1991). Many residents enjoy cuddling and petting animals, which they find calming and soothing. Choosing the most appropriate animal for the resident is important. Policies and procedures for pet programs should be in place prior to the first visit. Numerous organizations, including natural history museums, animal protection leagues, and Pets on Wheels, may sponsor programs that bring pets and nursing home residents together. In some areas, zoos also work with local nursing homes, bringing reptiles into the facilities. For information on animal-assisted therapy, readers can contact the Delta Society (P.O. Box 1080, Renton, WA 98057-1080).

Diversional Activities

Diversional activities are designed to reduce agitation and redirect energies for short periods of time. They can be initiated by any staff member. Residents may enjoy rummaging through a "junk" drawer, a woman's purse, or a man's tool box. Magazines or theme books can be given to residents to glance at during slow periods of the day. Building blocks or simple puzzles can become a joint project for residents, staff, and visitors.

COGNITIVE AND EDUCATIONAL ACTIVITIES

Cognitive and educational activities scheduled into the therapeutic recreation and activities program facilitate intellectual stimulation and empower personal growth. These programs keep residents involved in the world around them, provide a sense of purpose, and allows the residents to draw on past experiences. Additional objectives are shown in Table 12.8.

Discussion groups, current event sessions, letter writing, educational series, living room learning sessions, community service projects, and participating in games are all examples of cognitively stimulating activities. Guidelines for conducting cognitive and educational activities are shown in Table 12.9.

Cards, Board Games, and Bingo

Residents enjoy the fun, challenge, and competition of cards, board games, and bingo. Card games provide diversion and entertainment. Favorite card games for older adults include Uno, solitaire, concentration, black jack, poker, rummy, and pinochle. Large print and jumbo-size cards are available for residents with visual impairments. Trivial Pursuit, Wheel of Fortune, Scrabble, Memory, Pictionary, and Go to the Head of the Class can be adapted for nursing home residents. There are also many variations to bingo, such as color bingo, shape bingo, music bingo, and name bingo.

Theme Books

Making theme books devoted to a particular theme or subject can be enjoyable for older people. Theme books can be made from magazines, cards, newspapers, wallpaper, and wrapping paper. Suggested topics include: babies, flowers, animals, food, colors, holi-

Table 12.8. Objectives of cognitive and educational activities

Enhance opportunities for sharing knowledge and experience.
Assist residents to learn new things.
Allow for creative outlets.
Help maintain independence.
Promote self-confidence and feelings of self-worth.
Foster opportunities for ego satisfaction.
Cultivate new skills and interests.
Encourage the use of previous skills by providing continuing educational opportunities.
Stimulate group discussions for exchange of opinions and social interactions.
Provide work tasks to maintain abilities, use skills, and feel useful.
Stimulate awareness of the physical environment.

Table 12.9. Guidelines for conducting cognitive and educational activities

Plan activities to keep residents mentally alert.

Structure activities to meet the functional level of the resident.

Plan programs around simple and retained skills.

Increase difficulty of tasks by sequencing or building on successes.

Foster a warm and relaxed atmosphere to encourage interaction and participation.

Encourage residents who appear reluctant to participate.

Respect each resident's right to participate.

Facilitate discussion by reflecting on life experiences.

Survey the residents periodically throughout the year to develop ideas for future educational programs.

Place residents so that all can see and hear if audiovisual equipment is used.

Use various forms of media to enhance all the senses.

Use a microphone or sound system when lecturers are scheduled.

days, and advertisements. Once the theme books are completed, they should be made accessible to all staff, family, and friends to use in conversation with the residents.

Living Room Learning Movie Series

Video cassettes and 16-mm films can be shown to create a classroom atmosphere. Numerous film and television series, such as "Ascent of Man," "The Civil War," and "Roots," can be borrowed from public libraries, video stores, and public television stations. Large screen projection is recommended to recreate the atmosphere of a movie theater. A discussion period can be conducted after viewing an educational movie or video.

Discussion Groups

Current events, television shows, and reminiscing about previous experiences are often successful topics for group discussion. Favorite holidays, nicknames, vacations of long ago, and fashion are also appropriate topics. A more complete list of topics can be found in the *Complete Handbook of Activities and Recreational Programs for Nursing Homes* (1981), by Linda Hastings. BIFOLKAL KITS, manufactured by Bifolkal Productions, offers educational and reminiscent programs with themes such as "Remembering Train Rides," "Remembering The Depression," and "Remembering Fashion." These educational kits can be borrowed from many library systems.

Cooking and Food Sampling

Activities involving food are particularly popular in nursing homes. Tasting homemade foods and participating in the making of the food can be enjoyable as well as socially and physically beneficial. Residents socialize, share memories, use retained skills, and perhaps learn new skills when participating in culinary groups.

The variety of foods that can be made in the nursing home ranges from Jell-O to complete meals. Many foods can be prepared without cooking or baking and thus may not require a kitchen. Small kitchen appliances, such as a toaster oven, ice cream maker, bread maker, and sandwich maker can be used.

Community Service Projects

Folding newsletters, stuffing envelopes, making decorations and placemats for theme days, and assembling mailings for other organizations are all examples of community service activities. Other activities include: delivering flowers, mail, and birthday gifts; and packaging craft items for a fundraising sale. Community service projects give residents a sense of contributing to the community and provide an enhanced feeling of self-worth. Recognizing the residents for their volunteer efforts is an important component of community service activities.

Work-Oriented Activities

Work-oriented activities draw on past experiences and empower residents with a sense of accomplishment and purpose. Suggestions for such activities include: assisting with setting the table, watering plants, calling bingo, collating papers, assisting in the gift shop or craft room, and pushing a hospitality cart.

Solo Activities

Activities that are done alone rather than in groups can provide mental stimulation and can channel excess energy into success-oriented programs. Examples of activities that can be done alone include: playing cards, working on puzzles, stuffing envelopes, stringing beads, wrapping gifts, rolling yarn, folding fabric, and pounding aluminum cans for recycling. Solo activities may be arranged to fill in time between group activities or may be the primary means of activity involvement for individuals who refuse group participation.

CREATIVE EXPRESSION ACTIVITIES

Creative activities provide outlets for the expression of feelings and moods, stimulate creative talents, and reinforce feelings of self-worth and satisfaction. Participation of residents in creative arts may increase socialization, raise spirits, capture attention, and provide opportunities for the release of tension and aggression. Painting, music, dance, drama, art, crafts, and gardening are examples of creative expression activities. Both cognitively intact and cognitively impaired residents can benefit from creative expression. Program objectives and guidelines for conducting creative expression activities are provided in Tables 12.10 and 12.11, respectively.

Music Appreciation

Music is a form of communication. It sends a message without words, creates a mood, and can energize or soothe. The opportunity to listen to music can be provided in many forms. Residents may attend concerts in the community or in the nursing home, or listen to the radio or recorded music. Choirs, pianists, accordion players, and guitarists may provide live performances for residents and staff. Audio cassettes, records, videotapes, and televised performances are all appropriate for use with groups or individuals.

Sing-a-Longs

Sing-a-longs are extremely popular in nursing homes. Group singing can be done informally, in impromptu songfests, or formally, in organized choirs. Residents with poor short-term memory often recall the lyrics to popular songs of an earlier era and delight in group sing-a-longs.

Rhythm Bands

Instruments for rhythm bands can be constructed or purchased. Harmonicas, kazoos, rhythm sticks, washboards, shakers, maracas, spoons, tambourines, pie tins, recorders, and drums can all be used in the band. The addition of instruments promotes active participation of residents in the music and encourages movement.

Table 12.10. Objectives of creative expression activities

Promote feelings of self-worth, self-respect, and dignity.
Allow a temporary escape from reality of one's situation.
Provide an outlet for expressions of feelings such as anxiety, joy, faith, and fear.
Build feelings of fellowship and kinship.
Provide an acceptable outlet for fantasizing.
Stimulate sensory awareness through movement and art.

Table 12.11. Guidelines for conducting creative expression activities

Adopt a multisensory approach when incorporating music and dance.

Select music that will appeal to the residents.

Structure groups based on the size of the room and the types of residents involved.

Allow space between residents to accommodate dance movements.

Use nontoxic supplies when creating art projects.

Experiment with various media.

Use judgment when selecting supplies; small objects can be mistaken for food items.

Select craft or art projects that are simple enough to be completed by the residents.

Allow enough time to complete projects.

Use a nonjudgmental, supportive approach when encouraging creative expression in art.

Dances

Traditional and modern dance activities can be incorporated into many programs. Broadway, classical, and Big Band dance music are suggested for dance movements. The use of music and rhythmic movements as part of exercise was examined earlier in this chapter. As a creative outlet, residents should be encouraged to move to the music in their own ways and to use the essence of the dance to foster self-expression. Through arm movements, upper body sway, and wheelchair gliding, even chairbound residents can participate in dance activities. Holiday or theme dances, where residents, staff, and families are encouraged to dress festively, can become annual social events in the nursing home.

Arts and Crafts

Many arts and crafts ideas and resources are available at the public library. The key is to adapt projects to meet the needs and interests of the residents. Arts and crafts projects should be success oriented. For nursing home residents, this means selecting projects that can be completed in a relatively short period of time, before the resident becomes restless. Uncomplicated projects should be chosen, and specific instructions should be given. Simple arts and crafts projects, prepackaged with instructions, supplies, and samples, can be made available on the units so that residents are occupied while passing time waiting for other major events of the day. Staff, volunteers, families, and visitors can be encouraged to initiate simple projects with individual residents or small groups of residents. This involvement will provide nursing and allied health professionals additional opportunities for observing the residents, and will provide diversion by filling unoccupied time with meaningful activities. This is particularly critical for residents who are at risk of falling and are no longer restrained.

Other Means of Creative Expression

Drama and nature activities are other types of programs that can be planned to facilitate creative expression. By offering a variety of such activities, a facility is more likely to maintain resident interest and involvement and meet the needs of many residents.

SOCIAL ACTIVITIES

The need for innovative recreational programming in long-term care facilities is essential to promote socialization and maintain the quality of life of all residents. Social programs serve as alternatives to restraints because they can reduce isolation, depression, withdrawal, wandering, and agitation. Examples of social activities include: special theme meals, restaurant nights, deli days, ice cream socials, picnics, coffee klatches, and happy hours. Such activities are success oriented, motivating, and undemanding. Residents can be active or passive participants in these types of activities. Social activities facilitate interaction and forge a common bond among residents, staff, families, volunteers, and visitors. Objectives of social activities and guidelines for conducting such activities are shown in Tables 12.12 and 12.13, respectively.

Food Socials

Food is often used as an enticement to motivate residents, who enjoy extra opportunities to eat and drink. Food socials are activities that are structured around specific refreshments, used as a medium to increase socialization among residents. Ice cream, coffee cake, donuts, alcoholic and nonalcoholic drinks, hors d'oeuvres, canapes, chips and snacks, cookies, and cheese and crackers can be served at food socials.

Special Meal Events

Most residents have limited opportunities to visit restaurants. The illusion of a restaurant can be brought into the facility, however. Banquets, deli cafe, international restaurant night, and theme meals offer the therapeutic recreation and activities staff oppor-

Table 12.12. Objectives of social activities

Maintain and/or restore social skill.
Provide opportunities for social interaction.
Improve or maintain interpersonal relationships.
Provide a change of environment.
Enhance the resident's feelings of self-esteem and increase feelings of self-worth.
Reinforce appropriate behaviors while utilizing social skills in a social setting.
Decrease boredom.
Build group cohesiveness and sense of community.

tunities to work with other departments and to involve residents in the planning process. A theme can be used to coordinate the food and decorations. Special meal events can be held to celebrate holidays (e.g., Valentine's Day, St. Patrick's Day, Mother's Day, Father's Day), or they can focus on a particular theme (e.g., country fair, Oktoberfest, the Roaring Twenties) or cuisine (e.g., Chinese, Italian, Hawaiian, deli).

Men's and Ladies' Clubs

Groups segregated by sexes often facilitate freer conversation and increased socialization. The groups can be developed according to theme, projects, topics, or food. For example, since men often enjoy talking about sports, Mondays are a good day for rehashing Sunday's games. Friday "betting circles" provide opportunities for prospec-

Table 12.13. Guidelines for conducting social activities

Limit the size of the group when planning for residents with particular behavior problems, such as wandering or agitation.
Allow distance in seating other residents around an agitated resident.
Place residents who wander closer to the leader so that they can be easily redirected.
Make attempts to pair residents who are compatible.
Encourage the buddy system by pairing an alert, well-oriented resident with a less capable resident; one resident's calming manner may positively affect an agitated resident.
Place few demands in order to foster communication and social interaction.
Recognize various forms of participation (i.e., passive and active).
Validate each individual's needs and respect each person's right to participate as he or she chooses.

tive analysis of the week's games. Women may enjoy discussing current events, books they are reading, or their families.

Special Events

Special events, such as a Mardi Gras party or a casino night, provide residents the opportunity to stretch their imaginations and involve families, staff, and volunteers. These activities bring in the community, build excitement and enthusiasm among residents and staff, allow for an element of surprise, and allow a change of routine. Kentucky Derby Day, Haunted Hallway, Gingerbread with Santa, and Night at the Races are a few examples of special events appropriate for long-term care facilities.

Intergenerational Activities

Intergenerational activities bring together the young and the old and enrich the lives of all who participate. Intergenerational activities can involve family members (i.e., children and grandchildren of the residents) or unrelated young people (e.g., preschool children from a neighboring day care center). Both the residents and the children who participate in such activities derive pleasure from the experience. One way to bring generations together is to host school children of all ages at holiday times or on a regular basis throughout the year. Family members can be invited to carnivals and Mother's and Father's Day events. Encouraging residents to volunteer at neighboring schools, hospitals, and libraries also provides the opportunity for contact with younger people.

Outings

Field trips and outings provide a variety of experiences, offer a change of environment, and make life more meaningful and enjoyable for residents. Trips offer residents opportunities for interesting and varied interactions within the community, and help maintain the sense of continuity with the community. Residents usually take more interest in their personal appearance when going on outings. Examples of appropriate outings include: visiting another nursing home for a program; attending a community dance or theater production; going out to a meal at a restaurant; attending a prom for senior citizens; participating in a citywide nursing home Olympics; and visiting local churches, libraries, or schools to participate in special programs.

Field trips may not be appropriate for all residents. A resident who wanders requires close supervision if taken on a field trip. An agitated, disruptive resident's behavior may be problematic in any public area.

THE ROLE OF ACTIVITIES IN
A RESTORATIVE CARE ENVIRONMENT

This chapter has described a variety of activities that can be used as alternatives to physical and chemical restraints. As with other alternatives, the key to successful intervention is individualized assessment. No one group of activities has been found to be the most effective alternative to restraints for a particular type of resident. All wanderers do not enjoy arts and crafts. All agitated residents are not calmed by soft music. Each resident must be assessed in terms of abilities, disabilities or problems, preferences, interests, and past experiences, and encouraged to attend activities that most appropriately meet his or her needs.

In addition to serving as alternatives to restraints, therapeutic activities must incorporate and be incorporated into a total philosophy of restorative care. Therapeutic activities foster a restorative care philosophy by refocusing all activities toward maximizing independent functioning. For example, movement and exercise can be included in even the most sedentary of activities. Even a 5-minute stretch break during a long passive activity can help to improve the attention span of older residents. Encouraging and assisting residents who are able to walk all or part of the way to activities reinforces a restorative approach.

Therapeutic activities are incorporated into a total restorative care philosophy through an interdisciplinary approach to activities and a recognition that activities can take place throughout the day, not just at designated program times. An interdisciplinary approach involves all departments in facilitating and providing activities for residents. Therapeutic recreation and activities departments should be invited to take a more active role in sharing information, making resources available, and providing training to facilitate activities as alternatives to restraints.

Nursing assistants are critical to activities and should be involved in team meetings at which residents' needs are identified and plans of care developed. When activities are viewed as an integral component of the residents' plan of care and nursing assistants are included in developing that plan of care, nursing assistants will be more likely to encourage residents to participate in activities.

Volunteers, families, visitors, and nursing assistants can be taught to initiate individual and group activities throughout the day. Puzzles, cards, theme books, beach balls, and beauty supplies are some items that can be stored on units and made available throughout the day to individuals who have a few spare moments or an entire afternoon to spend with residents. Lag times, such as time waiting for meals or waiting to go to sleep are excellent times to initiate such activities. Filling waiting moments with activities that help to improve function or distract a person who is agitated, restless, or forgetful of reminders not to walk unassisted supports the restorative care philosophy.

CONCLUSION

Therapeutic activities in a nursing home can benefit the physical, cognitive, social, and emotional well-being of all residents. In a restorative care philosophy, all residents have the right to function at their maximum ability, regardless of impairment, while developing, maintaining, and expressing an appropriate leisure lifestyle.

Since the Omnibus Budget Reconciliation Act (OBRA) of 1987, the direction of therapeutic recreation and activities has been to enhance quality of life while supporting a restraint-free environment. A resident-appropriate and success-oriented activities program raises residents' self-esteem by focusing on abilities rather than impairments. Working with other staff members through an interdisciplinary approach, staff will find that activities can be one of the best alternatives to restraints and may improve the functional level of the residents as well.

Therapeutic recreation and activities interventions can be used to lessen agitation, to reduce tension, and to redirect energy. Activities also provide cognitive stimulation, an outlet for creative expression, and opportunities for social interaction. All of the above are important to maintaining the quality of life of residents in long-term care facilities.

REFERENCES

Barry, H.C. (1986). Exercise prescriptions for the elderly. *American Family Physician, 34*(3), 155–162.

Benison, B., & Hogstel, M.O. (1986). Aging and movement therapy:Essential interventions for the immobile elderly. *Journal of Gerontological Nursing, 12*(12), 8–16.

Blakeslee, J. (1989, December). *Individualized and environmental alternatives to restraints.* Paper presented at the conference Untie the Elderly, Columbia, MD.

Fleischmann, B., & Van Hala, B. (1982). It's not just bingo: Recreation in long term care facilities. *The Sounding Board* (publication of Ohio Parks and Recreation Associates), Spring, 5–6.

Glickstein, J.K. (1991). The golden key club. *Geriatric Care and Rehabilitation, 5*(1), 1–8.

Hastings, L. (1981). *Complete handbook of activities and recreational programs for nursing homes.* Englewood Cliffs, NJ: Prentice Hall.

Hopkins, D.R., Murrah, B., Hoeger, W., & Rhodes, R.C. (1990). Effect of low-impact aerobic dance on the functional fitness of elderly women. *The Gerontologist, 30*(2), 189–192.

Koroknay, V., Werner, P., Cohen-Mansfield, J., & Braun, J. (1991). A nursing administered walking program in the nursing home. *The Gerontologist, 31*(11), 219.

Norman, G.M., & Gibbs, J.A. (1991). Why walk when you can ride? *Journal of Gerontological Nursing, 17*(8), 29–33.

Orr, L.H., & DeProspero, R. (1991). Interdisciplinary mobility enhancement/immobility prevention program. *The National Conference of Gerontological Nurse-Practitioners Newsletter, 30.*

Weisberg, J., & Pack, M. (1991). Hannah Katz's resident tabby. *Geriatric Nursing, 12*(3), 117–118.

Weiss, J., (1988). *The feeling great! wellness program for older adults,* a special issue of *Activities, Adaptation and Aging,* Vol. 12 (3/4). New York: Haworth Press.

Chapter 13

Behavior Management Assessment

Renee Clermont and Jeanne R. Samter

It is estimated that half of all residents living in nursing homes suffer from cognitive impairment, and that 70% of these residents—or about one-third of all nursing home residents—exhibit some forms of disruptive behaviors (Ray, Taylor, Lichtenstein, & Meador, 1992). Central to being able to deal with these behaviors is the ability to assess them. This need has grown since 1987, when the Omnibus Budget Reconciliation Act (OBRA), limiting the use of physical and chemical restraints, was passed. Following the passage of OBRA, the Health Care Financing Administration (HCFA) reaffirmed the right of nursing home residents to be "free of any physical restraints imposed or psychoactive drugs administered for purposes of discipline or convenience and not required to treat the resident's medical symptoms" (HCFA, 1989). The greater scrutiny now associated with the use of restraints means that behavioral assessment is now more important than ever.

A behavior management assessment is much like good detective work. Like an investigation, an assessment examines the problem from several perspectives, and involves all those with a stake in the problem—including family and staff. In a facility with a restorative care philosophy, the behavior management assessment is based on the principle of fostering residents' independence and autonomy. Solutions to problem behavior are determined in terms of what is best for the resident; the risks associated with a particular approach to the problem are weighed against the benefits to the resident before a particular intervention is selected.

Under certain, narrowly defined circumstances, restraints may be used as treatment. The American Association of Homes for the Aging (Collopy, 1992) recommends the use of restraints only when they are needed "to ensure the resident's or other's safety and with a written physician order specifying the duration and circumstances." Before restraints are used, however, all residents must be assessed. The assessment begins with the designation of one person to integrate all the assessment data that will be collected. Other professionals, including both staff members and outside consultants who will be involved in the assessment, should also be identified.

For all behavior problems, the assessment must cover four important areas: 1) medications, 2) physical illnesses, 3) functional problems, and 4) history of psychiatric illness, shown in Table 13.1.

COLLECTING INFORMATION

A behavior management assessment begins by identifying the resident's behavior as clearly and precisely as possible. Three main sources of information—the resident's medical record; the facility's records on the resident; and interviews with the resident, with staff, and with family members—are available to caregivers.

Examining the Resident's Medical Record

A resident's medical record is an invaluable source of information that may reveal patterns in behavior, responses to treatment and medication, and past use of medications. Table 13.2 includes a list of questions that the clinical nurse specialist or other professional re-

Table 13.1. Areas that need to be covered by a behavior management assessment

Medications used by resident
    Changes to medications, including increases and decreases of dosages and additions of new medications

    Toxic responses to existing medications related to infection and cumulative effects

Physical illnesses experienced by resident
    Acute conditions, including infections and changes in vital signs

    Chronic conditions, including degeneration and exacerbation of conditions

Functional problems experienced by resident
    Permanent admission to long-term care

    Recent change to a new unit

    Changes in family system, such as deaths, births, divorces, and resident's perception of changes in the family

Psychiatric illnesses experienced by resident

Table 13.2. Questions to answer when reviewing the resident's medical record as part of the behavior management assessment

1. When was the resident admitted to the facility?
2. What was the reason for the resident's admission to the facility?
3. Does the resident have a psychiatric diagnosis?
4. Did the resident have any psychiatric interventions prior to his or her admission? If so, what were the results?
5. Has the resident undergone psychological testing? If so, what did the testing reveal?
6. When did the resident's disturbed behavior begin?
7. Were there any indications of disturbed behavior patterns prior to the resident's admissions?
8. What has been done about the behavior in the past?
9. What medications, especially antipsychotics, sleeping pills, or antidepressants, have been prescribed for the resident?
10. Has the resident received somatic medications, such as antiarrythmic betablockers or other medications, that have depressive properties?
11. Does anyone in the family have durable power of attorney?
12. What are the resident's daily patterns (e.g., does the resident wake up early or sleep late? Which meal does the resident prefer?)?
13. Are any strengths that may allow the care team to work with the resident more effectively noted in the medical record?

sponsible for the assessment should answer when examining the resident's medical records.

Examining Facility Records

The facility's records are another valuable source of information. These records include the incident report, the 24-hour report, the record of in-house daily changes, the postadmission conference (PAC), the psychotropic drug review, and screening assessments. All of these records can help the caregiver identify problems or track patterns, and should be examined carefully as part of the assessment.

The *incident report* is completed only when an unusual incident, such as a fall or an assault, results from a resident's problem behavior. Incident reports are useful means of monitoring significant patient care problems, particularly in large facilities.

The *24-hour report* can also help keep track of residents' disturbing or violent behaviors. A quick review of these reports after a weekend or holiday can provide the caregiver with an overview of any behavior management problems that a resident may have experienced.

The *record of in-house daily changes* is a written documentation of the transfer of residents within the facility or from the facility to a hospital. It also indicates room changes and deaths on the unit. Some of these changes may cause residents to experience stress. The record of in-house changes can alert the staff that a resident's new symptoms of agitation or depression may be related to these changes.

The *post-admission conference (PAC)* is a useful way to gather information for a comprehensive assessment of a resident. In this conference, held within the first week of the resident's admission, the family is invited to meet with all members of the treatment team. Each member of the team discusses with the family the initial assessment and the care plan designed to help the resident achieve his or her highest level of functioning. Team members solicit the comments and recommendations of the family and the resident, as well as any pertinent background information regarding the resident's previous life patterns and daily routines. Review of this record can help in assessing a resident for behavior management.

The *psychotropic drug review* is an important and informative way to track the progress of residents who are taking psychotropic drugs. The review of psychotropic drugs is generally done by the psychiatrist, physician, nurse, pharmacist, and/or social worker, with input from the nurse manager or charge nurse. This review allows the effectiveness or lack of effectiveness of the resident's medications to be evaluated. Following the review, dosages are often changed or drugs discontinued altogether.

Screening tools help enormously in assessing changes in a resident's behavior. Many facilities use a screening tool at the time of the resident's admission. This is a helpful practice that can augment other assessments to determine a resident's baseline functioning. The most widely used of the many instruments available are Folstein's Mini-Mental State Exam (MMSE) (Folstein, Folstein, & McHugh, 1975) and Yesavage's Geriatric Depression Scale (GDS) (Yesavage et al., 1983). Both are quick and easy to use.

Interviewing the Resident, the Staff, and Families

Central to understanding the resident's behavior are interviews with the resident, with staff who work with the resident, and with the resident's family. At many facilities, a geropsychiatric clinical nurse specialist conducts the interviews. Facilities that do not have access to such a professional should rely on a charge nurse or nurse manager rather than on outside consultants, since outside consultants will not be available to discuss the resident's behavior with members of all shifts and all departments.

Interviewing the Resident   Determining what a problem behavior means to the resident is a significant factor in the assessment that is sometimes overlooked. Once the behavior that the assessment will target has been identified, the resident should be interviewed to determine his or her own perception of the behavior, and to allow the person conducting the interview to observe the behavior. While the assessor is with the resident, he or she should keep the following questions in mind:

1. What triggered the behavior?
2. What changes may have taken place in the resident's environment?
3. Who is in the resident's immediate environment?
4. What is that person doing?
5. What else is going on in the resident's life?

Interviewing Staff Who Work with the Resident   Sometimes a resident repeats the behavior throughout the day, making direct observation easy. In other instances, only a few staff members may have observed the behavior in its most extreme form. It is thus important to interview as many staff on as many different shifts as possible.

The primary nursing assistant, who is most familiar with the resident, is crucial to the assessment. He or she may be the first to perceive sudden changes in a resident's behavior. The observations of auxiliary staff are also important, and may enhance the accuracy of the assessment. Some questions that may be helpful in conducting the interviews with staff are shown in Table 13.3. A written log of each interview should be kept.

Table 13.3.   Questions to ask during staff interviews as part of behavior management assessment

1. Which behavior is most troublesome for the resident and the staff?
2. How troublesome is the behavior?
3. Who is most bothered by the behavior?
4. When did this behavior start?
5. How often does this behavior occur?
6. When does this behavior tend to occur?
7. What strategies have been used in the past to manage this behavior?
8. Did any of these strategies work?
9. Has the resident's family been consulted?
10. What does the family say about the resident's behavior?
11. Did the family offer any strategies that were successful in coping with this behavior?

Not everyone observes a behavior the same way, and not everyone ascribes the same meaning to particular behaviors. Hence, the person or persons who noticed the behavior problem should be identified by name in the assessment. This information may reveal areas in which staff development is needed. If, for example, only one staff member or one group of staff members consistently describes a particular resident as problematic, the supervisor or director of nursing may want to look into why this resident's behavior is perceived differently by these staff. Where certain staff consistently report a particular kind of problem behavior, the supervisor or director of nursing may want to investigate whether or not these staff are overly sensitive to a particular behavior.

The following case study highlights the importance of the interview process in data collection:

Mrs. Talbott, an 87-year-old resident, was referred to the geropsychiatric clinical nurse specialist for a room change evaluation. Staff, particularly the evening shift staff, were suffering burnout as a result of the heavy care requirements demanded by Mrs. Talbott, whose difficult behavior made caring for her trying.

Before moving Mrs. Talbott to another unit, staff were interviewed as part of a behavior management assessment. Although Mrs. Talbott's primary nursing assistant and other staff from both shifts reported difficult behaviors, none of the staff, including those on the night shift, really wanted Mrs. Talbott transferred.

All of those interviewed corroborated the report that the resident's behavior was much worse during the evening shift. Management strategies were thus designed to help the evening staff cope. The staff examined the resident's medications, treatments, and care needs, and shifted the responsibility for as many of these needs as possible to members of the day shift. The nurse manager and the geropsychiatric clinical nurse specialist then conducted care conferences with members of the evening shift to determine whether the changes had been effective. When they determined that the changes had been effective, the request for the resident's transfer was cancelled.

Interviewing Family Members An interview with the resident's family can help the caregiver in several ways. First, the family can provide information on the resident's earlier behavior patterns. A resident whose life pattern has been to "act out" whenever he or she needs attention will continue this behavior in the nursing home.

Second, the family can inform caregivers of any changes that may have occurred in the family system. A *nodal event* is an unusual happening, such as a death, a birth, or a serious illness, that affects a family system. Nodal events may precipitate a resident's behavior problems. Emotional connections in families run deep, and disturbances in the family may affect the resident, causing him or her to engage in disturbed behavior. Residents are often distressed to learn that the family has concealed a nodal event, such as the death or marriage of someone close to them. They may be disturbed to learn that their families have chosen not to tell their friends and relatives of their permanent move to the nursing home. Only by talking to family members would staff be aware of these sources of stress.

Strained relationships with a significant family member may create an emotional disturbance that gives rise to a behavior problem. Sometimes the fact that other residents have visitors will make a resident feel more acutely the absence of his or her own family members. The resident may feel abandoned or rejected by the lack of visitors. Such feelings bring sadness, and if they are prolonged they may provoke depressions. By interviewing family members, staff can uncover underlying family problems that may account for the resident's behavior problems.

Describing the Environment

A description of conditions in the facility should also be included in the assessment of the resident's behavioral problems. Some conditions that may affect resident behavior are understaffing, ongoing preparations for field trips, or shift changes. Other factors that may exacerbate a resident's inappropriate behavior include changes in the movement patterns and tones of voice of some of the other residents. Staff members may also upset residents by moving too hastily, speaking too loudly, and using the telephone or intercom.

USING FLOW SHEETS TO DOCUMENT THE RESIDENT'S BEHAVIOR

Flow sheets may be useful in monitoring a resident's behavior problems on a short-term (i.e., 24-hour) basis. The geropsychiatric clinical nurse specialist uses two types of flow sheets. The *behavioral assessment form* is used when a nurse manager calls for help in assessing a resident with several behavior problems. The nurse manager may want to begin by working with the staff to identify problem behaviors. One informative way of doing so is to have the nurse manager compile a list ahead of time to see if that list matches the list prepared by the staff.

The flow sheet itself should include the resident's name and an evaluation of his or her behavior. A sample unit behavioral assessment form is shown in Figure 13.1. The form should indicate the frequency of the behavior and the duration of each episode. It is also useful to note the shift during which the resident most often engages in the behavior and the rank of importance the staff member gives to this behavior.

If a resident has many behavior problems, the form should focus on the most troublesome while listing all of the problem behaviors. These should be listed in order of difficulty involved in managing them, with the most difficult problems listed last. The psychology that underlies behavior management is that success breeds success. If staff members begin with some of the easier problems, their confidence will grow.

The *individual resident flow sheet* is used to obtain a clear picture of the frequency, duration, and degree of the resident's problem behavior. At times, behavior problems are elusive. Often, they reflect the biased perceptions of the observer. An individual 24-hour behavioral assessment form, a sample of which is shown in Figure 13.2, helps to separate the facts from the feelings. A good flow sheet also provides ample space to document any environmental factors that may have influenced the resident's behavior.

ANALYZING THE INFORMATION OBTAINED

Once all information on the resident has been collected and documented, the next step is to determine realistic goals for behavior change. To do so, the assessor needs to describe outcomes that reinforce the resident's behavior by asking:

1. What does the resident get from this behavior?
2. How do others respond?
3. What does the resident do after the caregiver responds to the behavior?
4. What triggers may be eliminated or modified?
5. What reinforcers may be eliminated?
6. What reinforcers may be introduced to help the resident behave more appropriately?
7. What new triggers might prompt new behaviors?

After collecting and analyzing the information, the staff can make a decision regarding the need to call in a consultant. The more information that has been gathered, the more effectively the staff will be able to work with the consultant.

Date ____

Rank of behavior (from least difficult to most difficult)	Resident's name	Behavior	Frequency of behavior	Duration of behavior	Shift
4	Sophia Barnett	hits, bites, scratches	all showers Am pm & care	throughout	D,E
2	Sally Rodgers	refuses shower	every time offered	all day	D,E
1	Kay Dosier	finishes breakfast and goes back to bed	9 Am	'til lunch if allowed	D
3	Matilda Jacobs	curses, verbal abuse	worse during dressing	3-5 min.	D,E

Figure 13.1. Unit behavioral assessment form. Behaviors are ranked from least difficult to most difficult so that staff can deal with less difficult behaviors first.

231

Resident's name _____ Date _____

Frequency of behavior

Never	Less than once a week	Once or twice a week	Several times a week	Once or twice a day	Several times a day	A few times an hour
(1)	(2)	(3)	(4)	(5)	(6)	(7)

Duration of episode _____ minutes _____ hours

Degree   Mild (1)   Moderate (2)   Severe (3)

Time	Behavior	Frequency	Duration	Environment	Degree
12–1 AM					
1–2					
2–3					
3–4					
4–5					
5–6					
6–7					
7–8					
8–9					
9–10					

10–11

11–12 PM

12–1

1–2

2–3

3–4

4–5

5–6

6–7

7–8

8–9

9–10

10–11

11–12 AM

Figure 13.2. Individual 24-hour behavioral assessment form.

233

THE ROLE OF CONSULTANTS

Some of the larger facilities employ a psychiatric clinical nurse specialist to perform initial assessments, provide some of the mental health services offered, and coordinate the work of the mental health consultants. Some facilities contract for the consulting services of a psychiatrist or psychologist for a specified number of hours per week to assess the residents' behavior problems and make recommendations. In these facilities, it is recommended that the director of nursing, assistant director of nursing, or social worker coordinate the outside consultants.

The Role of the Psychiatrist

Psychiatrists contribute to the assessment process by diagnosing treatable mental disorders. They may review the resident's medications to determine whether drug interactions or other physical conditions are causing the behavior problem. They may offer suggestions for medication management, consult with staff physicians as needed, or provide individual weekly psychotherapy. They may also implement a routine review process of all psychotropic medications. Such a process is helpful in preventing acute behavioral problems that are related to psychotropic drug toxicity or side effects. It is also an effective means of monitoring the long-term use of psychotropic medications in the facility.

The Role of the Psychologist

Psychologists can administer psychological tests to determine which areas of a resident's functioning the staff might want to develop. Sometimes a resident's social graces mask severe deficits, leading staff to be less tolerant of aberrant behaviors because they think the resident is capable of better control. Psychological testing can reveal a resident's deficits as well as strengths.

Psychologists also provide one-on-one psychotherapy sessions and suggest strategies for helping other caregivers work with residents with cognitive impairment. They may be able to help staff focus on residents' strengths to best advantage.

Psychologists may also help the staff identify any environmental cues that may trigger residents' behavioral problems, as well as help develop methods of assessing the frequency and duration of residents' behaviors.

CASE STUDY

The complexity of assessing behavior problems cannot be overestimated. The following case study highlights some of the facets of the process.

In late October, the staff of the Plainview Home's moderate care unit decided that Mrs. Williams, a tiny, frail resident, needed a posey restraint to manage her falls and agitated behavior. Because the facility's policy stated that physical restraints could be used only as a last resort, the rehabilitation clinical nurse specialist was called in to perform an assessment.

It was painful to watch Mrs. Williams. Her gait was unsteady, her eyes were glassy, and she was unable to respond to the staff's constant urging that she ask for help whenever she wished to walk. The Vigil 88 alarm system on her wheelchair sounded regularly, notifying staff of her attempts to walk. At first glance, Mrs. Williams appeared to be in the state of agitation that staff of long-term care facilities recognize as the precursor to death.

The rehabilitation clinical nurse specialist invited the geropsychiatric clinical nurse specialist to collaborate on the assessment. She convened a care conference to communicate to the staff her position on the use of physical restraints and to offer them hope and encouragement that alternatives could be found. Only a few days earlier, she had requested that the psychiatrist review the use of Darvocet in the treatment of Mrs. Williams' back pain. She suspected that the Darvocet might be contributing to Mrs. Williams' agitation and loss of appetite. The psychiatrist concurred and discontinued the Darvocet.

During the care conference, the staff reviewed all of Mrs. Williams' medications. The geropsychiatric clinical nurse specialist recalled that the psychiatrist had increased her dose of Ritalin from 5 to 10 mg/day a few weeks earlier. She telephoned Mrs. Williams' primary physician to request that the Ritalin be discontinued.

She also noted that in July of the same year, the primary physician had increased Mrs. Williams' dose of nortriptyline from 50 to 75 mg at bedtime. She knew that 50 mg of nortriptyline was the maximum dose for a therapeutic response for this resident, and recalled that Mrs. Williams had developed paranoia and agitation when she had taken a higher dosage of this medication before. Within the week, the dose of Darvocet was tapered, the Ritalin was discontinued, and the dose of Nortriptyline was decreased to 50 mg at bedtime. Mrs. Williams then began walking with the aid of her walker. Her gait grew steady and her pace spritely. Her eyes sparkled and her appetite returned. The staff members were pleased with her progress and there was no further mention of the posey restraint.

The staff were pleased to observe that Mrs. Williams' condition improved when her medications were changed. The assessment was not complete, however, before the assessment team learned why the medications were prescribed for Mrs. Williams in the first place. By going back and examining Mrs. Williams' history, the team gained additional insight into her problems, improving their assessment skills for future cases.

CONCLUSION

The choice of interventions used to help residents achieve higher levels of functioning depends on the information gathered during the behavior management assessment. The gathering of this information is thus crucial.

In performing behavior management assessments, staff should maintain positive attitudes and should try to evaluate the results of the assessment objectively. Remaining positive will allow staff to try other intervention alternatives if and when the initial approach proves ineffective.

Staff may become discouraged by the amount of work involved in performing an assessment. Although the process does take time, inconsistent attempts to quiet a resident's disruptive behavior are also time consuming. The staff's energy and morale may drain away while the resident receives no real help in achieving his or her highest level of functioning. A good behavior management assessment may ultimately save staff time and improve the quality of care the resident receives.

REFERENCES

Collopy, B.J. (1992). *The use of restraints in long term care: The ethical issues.* White Paper, American Association of Homes for the Aging, Washington, DC.

Folstein, W.F., Folstein, S.E., & McHugh, P.R. (1975). Mini-mental state: A practical method for grading the cognitive state of patients for the clinician. *Journal of Psychiatric Research, 12,* 189–198.

Health Care Financing Administration. (1989). Regulations concerning use of restraints. *Federal Register, 54,* No. 21.

Med-Pass, Inc. (1990). *OBRA '87: Antipsychotic protocol handbook.* Dayton, OH: Med-Pass Incorporated.

Ray, W.A., Taylor, J.A., Lichtenstein, J.J., & Meador, K.G. (1992). The nursing home behavior problem scale. *Journal of Gerontology, 47*(1), 9–16.

Yesavage, J.A., Brink, T.L., Lum, O., Huang, O., Adey, M.B., & Leirer, V.O. (1983). Development and validation of a geriatric depression rating scale: A preliminary report. *Journal of Psychiatric Research, 17,* 37–49.

Chapter 14

Behavior Management Alternatives to Restraints

Jeanne R. Samter

Changes in the health care delivery system have meant that long-term care facilities now care for more residents with more illnesses and behavior problems. The most notable changes have been the use of cost-control measures, such as the diagnosis-related groups (DRGs) and the case-mix reimbursement system. The introduction of these measures has meant that hospital stays have become shorter and patients who need extended care are now admitted to long-term care facilities. The acuity level of residents of long-term care facilities has thus risen steadily during the 1980s and 1990s.

Older adults are especially vulnerable to the behavior problems often associated with debilitating illnesses. This may account for the very high rate of behavior problems among residents of long-term care facilities. As sicker older people are admitted to nursing homes, the demands on staff to understand mental health needs grow. Often, staff feel that they are not equipped to deal with residents with difficult behavioral problems, and use physical or chemical restraints with such residents out of a sense of frustration and perceived lack of alternatives.

PROBLEM BEHAVIOR DEFINED

The term *behavior problem* may be defined in several ways. Burgio, Jones, Butler, and Engel (1989) define behavior problems as disruptive behaviors. Others have defined behavior problems in terms of depression. Psychologists, psychiatrists, and nurses often define behavior problems in terms of agitation, or inappropriate verbal, vocal, or motor activity that cannot be explained by the resident's needs or confusion per se. Cohen-Mansfield (1986) has grouped agitated behaviors into three categories: 1) physically aggressive behavior, 2) verbally aggressive behavior, and 3) nonaggressive behavior. In her study of 107 long-term care facility residents, she found that 87 percent of the residents experienced one or more of these behaviors at least once a week.

Behavior problems often result from depression. Depression is a matter of concern to staff members when residents become gravely discontent or anxious, or when they lose their appetites, something that is often distressing to staff.

BEHAVIOR PROBLEMS AND PSYCHIATRIC DIAGNOSES

Rovner, Kafonek, Filipp, Lucas, and Folstein (1986) were the first to examine the relationship between behavioral problems and psychiatric diagnoses in older adults. A geriatric psychiatrist interviewed a random sample of intermediate-care residents and diagnosed them based on the *Diagnostic and Statistical Manual of Mental Disorders*, 3rd edition (DSM-III-R) criteria. He found that 94% of residents studied suffered from psychiatric disorders and that 76% demonstrated behavior problems.

In residents with psychiatric diagnoses, some problems, such as hallucinations and delusions, can be successfully treated with psychotropic drugs (see Chapter 10).

USING BEHAVIOR MANAGEMENT AS AN ALTERNATIVE TO RESTRAINTS

Because behavior problems have been so closely linked with restraint use, the goal of restraint reduction will probably remain elusive unless caregivers consider behavior management as an alternative approach. Not all behavior problems can be eliminated. However, caregivers can almost always find ways to help residents improve their level of functioning.

Ideally, a behavior management program should achieve several goals:

1. It must define what types of problems the facility's residents are experiencing. Assessments are the most effective means of identifying these problems.
2. It must implement the therapeutic interventions that will meet the residents' needs most successfully.
3. It must evaluate the effectiveness of its interventions.

The next several sections describe the basic elements of a behavior management program. Later in the chapter, more detailed information is provided on one very effective behavior management program, that of the Hebrew Home of Greater Washington.

Assessment: Defining the Problem

Identifying the behavior that the staff seeks to change is the first step in developing a behavior management plan. Before tackling assessment of behavior problems, the caregiver assigned this role should collect articles from the professional literature that address the behavior problems most frequently encountered in the facility. Reading about how others have dealt with behavior problems assures staff members that they are not alone in dealing with these problems. It can also stimulate creative thinking.

To help identify the target behavior, the facility should keep a log of all residents referred to the facility's mental health service for consultation. A sample log is shown in Figure 14.1. The log should include the resident's name and age, the date of the consultation, and the unit that referred the resident. Space should be left for a description of the resident's behavior and the proposed management strategy. Keeping such a log is simple and encourages follow-up of all consultations.

Once a log of all problem behaviors is compiled, categories of behaviors must be identified. Table 14.1 lists the categories of behavior management problems identified in the first year of the behavior management program's operation at the Hebrew Home of Greater Washington.

Implementation: Executing Therapeutic Interventions

The interventions examined in this section are interpersonal tools that are effective with all kinds of behavior problems. In working with residents with behavior problems, caregivers should:

1. Discuss the behavior problem with the resident.
2. Let the resident know exactly what behavior concerns the staff and why.
3. Determine how much the resident understands.
4. Show the resident the appropriate behavior for the situation that provokes his or her problem behavior.

Even residents with the most extreme dementia have moments of lucidity. Discussing the behavior problem with the resident is a way to include him or her in the care plan, and may reveal to the caregiver some of the factors that precipitate the behavior. It is also

Date	Unit	Resident's name and age	Description of problem behavior	Proposed management strategy	Effectiveness
27 July	3 East	Corine Berman	tearful & irritable c̄ others	Geriatric Depression Scale & 1:1 c̄ RN refer to Psych for MED EVAL	IMPROVED c̄ TALKING Tx GDS SCORE = 12 IMPROVED c̄ MEDICATION
27 July	5 North	Edith Klinger	bit nursing assistant Hole in sweater	Resident cognitively intact 1) Care conference 2) Physician to adjust Meds D/c 2010 ↑↑	STAFF VENTED RES IMPROVED
29 July	2 South	Ann Moran	tearful aphasic post stroke	Psych Eval Possible Med adjustment	IMPROVED BY SEPT. 12

Figure 14.1. Keeping a behavior management log, such as the one shown here, encourages follow-up of all consultations. The person completing the log describes the resident's behavior and records the proposed management strategy.

important to let cognitively intact residents know which of the other residents' behaviors are inappropriate.

Sometimes a word or simple gesture can eliminate mildly inappropriate behavior, as seen in the following case study:

> Mrs. Cohen, a resident with mild dementia, was explaining to the nurse that she was uncomfortable walking through the unit because she thought she had a problem with incontinence. Although Mrs. Cohen was in complete control of her bladder, she was convinced that she was incontinent, and the perception that she was wet caused her great distress. She tearfully lifted up her dress to show the nurse the pad she wore. The nurse gently patted her hand and helped her pull her dress down. Although the pad was dry, Mrs. Cohen again pulled up her dress and repeated her concern. The nurse smiled at her and whispered, "Even in this day and age, the ability to maintain a little mystery is still a good asset!" The nurse winked and again helped Mrs. Cohen pull her dress back down. Mrs. Cohen then smiled broadly. She did not lift up her dress again.

Working with Staff The most effective means of training staff to deal with difficult behavior is by way of example: *staff tend to follow the lead set by the person in charge.* Often, staff unconsciously imitate the leader's style and adopt the values and attitudes that they perceive are held by the supervisory staff. The way in which the staff leader reacts to behavior problems can thus set the tone for the entire unit. To instill the proper attitude among staff, the leader should convey the notion that a particular behavior is difficult, but that the team is able to tackle it.

Conducting interviews with staff about residents' behavior problems helps to identify staff perceptions of the problem, and lets staff know that their input is valued. Staff may also interpret being interviewed as a sign that their distress is finally being recognized. Interviews may help restore staff confidence that other alternatives can be tried, and may reinforce the staff member's feeling that he or she is a valuable member of the treatment team.

Care conferences can be effective tools for working with staff. The care conference is also an opportunity to present the resident's history to the staff. Learning what residents did earlier in their lives sometimes helps staff understand them better, thus enabling them to distinguish the rational from the emotional component of the behavior problem more effectively. Providing staff with information on a resident often helps to dissipate highly charged emotions concerning the problem, as the following case study illustrates:

Table 14.1.   Categories of behavior problems encountered at the Hebrew Home of Greater Washington

Psychomotor behaviors	Aggressive/antisocial behaviors	Verbally agitated behaviors
Goal-directed wandering	Scratching	Speaking loudly
Aimless wandering	Grabbing onto people or objects	Distorting own speech
Restlessness	inappropriately	Refusing to speak
Handling dressings (e.g., IV tubes)	Pushing	Speaking repetitively
Inappropriate robing and disrobing	Throwing objects	Inappropriately calling for help
Attempting to get to a different place	Destroying property	Verbally abusing staff or other residents
Hiding and hoarding objects	Making sexually aggressive advances	Making strange noises
Chewing objects	Exposing genitals	Screaming
Putting objects in mouth	Criticizing others	Making verbal sexual advances
Spitting	Provoking others	
Making noise (e.g., banging)	Urinating or defecating inappropriately	
	Biting	
	Hitting	
	Injuring self	
	Kicking	

Sleep-related behaviors	Suicide-related behaviors	Appetite-related behaviors
Difficulty falling asleep	Expressing wish to die	Decreased appetite
Early morning awakening	Attempting to commit suicide	Increased appetite
Disturbed sleep at night		Refusing food, water, or life support
Disturbed sleep during the day		treatment

Behaviors related to interest in the environment	Mood-related behaviors	Other behaviors
Failure to initiate conversation with others	Crying	Feeling guilty
Reduced level of activity	Feeling depressed	Wanting to be alone all of the time
	Flat affect	Somatic complaints without physiological basis
	Unstable affect	Decline in functional level without physiological basis
	Limited range of affect	Feelings of restlessness
		Decrease in ability to concentrate
		Evidence of psychomotor retardation

Perceptual distortions

Visual hallucinations
Auditory hallucinations
Paranoid delusions
Somatic delusions

Note: Categories are as per L.M. Struble & L. Sivertsen. (1987). Agitated behaviors in confused elderly patients. *Journal for Gerontological Nursing, 13*(11), 40–44; and J. Cohen-Mansfield. (1986). Agitated behaviors in the elderly: Preliminary results in the cognitively deteriorated. *Journal of the American Geriatrics Society, 34,* 722–727.

Six weeks after her admission to Meadowview, Mrs. Miller, a spry 95-year-old woman, became agitated. In an effort to control her perpetual movement and subsequent falls, the staff restrained Mrs. Miller in bed. No matter how she was restrained, however, she was able to slip out of her restraints and climb over the bed's siderails. Once she grabbed another resident's glasses and broke them. The staff at Meadowview became increasingly frustrated. Eventually, they requested a psychiatric consultation.

The geropsychiatric clinical nurse specialist held a care conference. "Mrs. Miller is a 95-year-old woman, admitted 6 weeks ago," she began. Immediately, a nursing assistant interrupted her. "Did you say 95? I thought she was 75!" Several other nursing assistants attending the conference chimed in. They, too, had believed that Mrs. Miller was 75 years old. "Well," volunteered one nursing assistant, "if she is 95, she can do whatever she wants!" Although the care conference continued, the new information about Mrs. Miller's age noticeably changed the staff's approach to the resident and promoted a positive shift in their attitude toward caring for her.

Staff should also receive as much information about the resident's family as possible. At times, nursing home staff feel that families simply dump their older members with behavior problems in nursing homes, and wonder, "If their families can't deal with them, how are we supposed to do so?" It is thus useful to have family members share with staff the struggles they have endured and the efforts they have made in trying to keep their relative at home. Once staff understand that families have tried hard to keep their older members out of the nursing home, they are often more compassionate in their approach to caregiving, as the case of Mr. Wiley illustrates:

Mr. Wiley was transferred from a moderate unit to a behavior management unit because he physically abused the nursing assistants shortly after he was admitted. Although he was confined to his bed, hard of hearing, and blind, he remained extremely strong, and the staff feared that he might injure them. Mrs. Wiley, a few years younger than her husband, has struggled for 2 years to provide the care required to keep her husband in their small apartment! The couple's two grown children, who live out of town, are supportive of their parents, but have other responsibilities that deter them from playing larger roles. In the 6 months prior to his admission to the facility, Mr. Wiley had grown increasingly abusive verbally and physically toward his wife. His physical care needs had increased and Mrs. Wiley found herself exhausted. On her husband's admission to the facility, she struggled to hold back tears. Upon learning of Mrs. Wiley's heroic efforts to manage her husband at home, the staff responded unanimously. "We'll take care of him now," they told a grateful wife.

Care conferences give the team the opportunity to develop a checklist of interventions for dealing with the resident's problems. Although each resident's behavior problem requires its own set of interventions, sometimes a care conference can help staff in dealing with a resident's unique needs.

Care conferences can also be used to teach staff how a particular disease syndrome relates to the resident's behavior management. One violent resident had normal-pressure hydrocephalus. Although he had a shunt in place, he suffered from dementia. His care conference focused on his medical problem and the functioning of the shunt. The question and answer session allowed much information on the resident's physical disability to be imparted to the staff, thus helping them to understand the resident better.

Follow-up care conferences provide staff with the opportunity to discuss successful interventions and to work together to develop changes to interventions that have not been effective. They enable staff to identify areas where further staff training is needed and to identify problem areas that should best be referred to an outside consultant.

Finally, care conferences can provide the nurse with an opportunity to hear the staff's concerns and to offer support when a resident behaves abusively toward a staff member. Failure to intervene in such a situation can lead to a cycle of abusive behavior. A psychiatric evaluation should be conducted whenever a resident behaves abusively toward the staff, since abusive behavior may stem from depression or from poor impulse control secondary to a stroke or psychiatric disorder. In some cases, psychological testing can help reveal the extent of a resident's cognitive abilities and deficits.

In summary, care conferences are useful vehicles for achieving the following:

1. Allowing staff to vent their feelings
2. Correcting misperceptions about the resident and his or her behavior
3. Teaching staff better ways of approaching a resident's problem behavior
4. Determining the level of support that staff feel they receive from the nurse manager

Working with Families Families can provide a wealth of information on a resident's behavior, and can often suggest helpful ways in which staff can manage the resident's behaviors. It is thus crucial that staff discuss the resident's behavior problems with family members.

Since medications often are prescribed for residents with behavior problems, it is essential to find out if the family is aware of any prior use of psychotropic drugs that may not have been documented in the resident's medical records. Family members may know if the resident has been treated with psychotropic drugs in the past, and how he or she responded.

Anxiety on the part of family members can often exacerbate a resident's behavior problems. Families thus need to be reassured, and a positive relationship established between staff and families. To establish such a relationship, caregivers should:

1. Establish a policy of holding a postadmission conference with families and all members of the treatment team within the first week after a resident's admission.

2. Engage families as allies by asking them how they managed the resident's behavior problems.

3. Instruct families to direct their concerns or questions to a designated contact person on the team.

4. Take the initiative in greeting anxious family members.

5. Meet with family members who are particularly anxious once a week for 20 minutes. These sessions should be held at the same time each week and the same members of the treatment team should be present at each meeting.

6. Encourage nursing assistants to redirect the concerns of angry family members to someone in a higher position of authority, such as the nurse manager.

7. Conduct follow-up meetings with families as needed to discuss a resident's progress or decline.

Developing a Care Plan

The nurse manager or charge nurse can use care conferences as an opportunity to gain the staff's assistance in developing a plan of action. Because the nursing assistants and other staff, not the consultants, are the ones who must work with the resident, a plan that comes from the staff has a far greater chance of working than does a plan that comes from an outside consultant. The case study that follows illustrates this point:

> After 6 months of dealing with Mr. Arnold, a physically abusive resident, staff members were becoming discouraged. The nurse manager requested that the geropsychiatric clinical nurse specialist present a series of classes on agitation, especially, physically abusive behavior.

In the classes, the nurse specialist discussed some of the standard methods for dealing with an agitated resident. She suggested having two staff members work with the resident simultaneously, and challenged the staff to develop their own plans for working with Mr. Arnold.

The staff responded positively to the specialist's lecture. In less than half an hour, the staff on the evening shift had drawn up a realistic eight-point plan. Two of the interventions targeted the times during which Mr. Arnold became the most difficult to deal with, namely, at mealtimes and bedtimes. The staff decided to try letting Mr. Arnold eat sandwiches, which he loved, rather than full-course meals in the evenings in order to accommodate his pacing. They also decided to prepare all of the other residents for bed before Mr. Arnold, thus allowing them more time to accommodate his needs.

Reducing the Level of Noise in the Facility

Managing the level of noise in the facility can be as important as managing the staff and residents. Noise can agitate residents with behavioral problems, and can annoy everyone on the unit, staff and residents alike.

Recognizing that a unit is too noisy is the responsibility of all staff members. Residents with dementia are unable to make judgments about how much noise they can tolerate. Many do not know to move away from a noisy place; others may be unable to move on their own, and thus are forced to wait until a staff member can remove them from a noisy area. Leaving residents with dementia in noisy areas can cause a chain reaction to set in whereby one resident's distressed cry causes other residents to cry.

Staff often contribute to the noise level on a unit, and may need to be reminded to speak softly and move in a relaxed manner. Awareness of the noise level can be encouraged by requesting staff input regarding ways in which to diminish the level of noise on the unit.

Establishing Interpersonal Relationships

The most effective tool in managing behavior problems is the staff's ability to establish and maintain positive, warm relationships with residents and their families. A primary nursing system is an invaluable means toward this end. In such a system, a nursing assistant is assigned to the same residents each day.

The quality of the relationships between staff and residents depends strongly upon the attitude staff bring to their jobs. Staff members who believe that any kind of improvement is impossible are unlikely to develop positive relationships with residents; staff members who believe that possibilities for improvement are vast are much more likely to do so. Many excellent nursing assistants seem to understand intuitively the importance of the need for control, privacy, and involvement with other people that older adults in nursing homes have. "I couldn't possibly go to the dining room without Joyce," a resident may say when the nursing assistant who usually cares for her has a day off. "Only she knows how to lay out my things properly. She always comes in early to help me before she helps anyone else."

Communicating with Difficult Residents

Several factors may complicate communication with older adults in long-term or acute care settings. Many older adults have sensory impairments that make hearing and/or seeing difficult. An increase in anxiety may interfere with the person's ability to concentrate.

Respectful communication is the foundation for initiating and maintaining relationships with others. Table 14.2 presents a list of communication strategies that are effective in helping prevent many kinds of behavior problems. All caregivers should learn and use these strategies for communicating with older patients and residents.

BEHAVIOR MANAGEMENT AT THE
HEBREW HOME OF GREATER WASHINGTON

The Hebrew Home of Greater Washington is a 550-bed long-term care facility with two separate buildings on one campus. The facility's behavior management program began with a staff of one full-time geropsychiatric clinical nurse specialist and consultants from a variety of other mental health professions. A half-time geropsychiatric clinical nurse specialist was added during the second year of the program.

The full-time geropsychiatric clinical nurse specialist serves as the Hebrew Home's mental health coordinator. Responsibilities include coordination of all mental health services in the facility, education of staff, consultation with caregivers, assessment of residents, and provision of mental health services to residents. The mental health coordinator maintains a record of all consultations with other health care professionals and follows up with the staff to evaluate the consultants' recommendations. The coordinator also provides crisis intervention and short-term therapy for residents who need those services and conducts preadmission visits with prospective residents at their homes or at the hospital, as needed.

Mental health services are available from licensed social workers and graduate social work students, as well as various consulting psychologists, psychiatrists, and a geropsychiatric fellows.

Table 14.2. Strategies for communicating with residents with dementia

1. Approach the resident gently, in an open, friendly, relaxed manner.
2. Speak slowly and softly in a low-pitched voice.
3. Listen to the resident. Your interest conveys respect and concern.
4. Begin each conversation by identifying yourself and calling the resident by name. ("Good morning, Mrs. Smith. I'm your nurse, Jane.")
5. Use short, specific, familiar words, and simple sentences. ("I'm Jane. I'm here to help with your bath.")
6. Use words the resident uses.
7. Give one direction or ask one question at a time.
8. Wait for an answer. If the resident does not respond, repeat the question.
9. Allow the resident frequent opportunities to join the conversation by speaking in short sentences rather than paragraphs and allowing the resident time to comment.
10. Stand or crouch about 3 feet from the resident so that you are face-to-face but not close enough to be threatening.
11. Maintain eye contact with the resident when you speak.
12. Refer to people by their names; avoid vague references to "him" or "her."
13. Help the resident if he or she seems to be groping for a word.
14. Many residents lose their train of thought mid-sentence. Repeat the resident's last words to help him or her continue talking.
15. Limit the number of "don't"s you use in conversation. State directions positively. ("I would like you to use your cane today, Mrs. Williams.")
16. Use facial expression and hand gestures to demonstrate your concern.
17. Use nonverbal praise. Nodding, smiling, patting, and touching seem to be effective ways of communicating with people who no longer seem to understand speech.
18. Provide immediate reassurance during the conversation if the resident indicates he or she is upset.
19. Respond to the resident's message rather than his or her words.
20. Show respect for the feelings the resident expresses, even if his or her facts are incorrect. ("It certainly would be unpleasant to have to eat burnt food!")
21. Try to avoid competing noise. Turn off the radio or television when you address the resident.
22. Watch for signs of restlessness and withdrawal, such as hand movements, looking away, or frowning. End the conversation if the resident seems unable to concentrate.
23. Demonstrate a self-care skill if a resident seems not to understand your directions.
24. Assume the resident can understand more than he or she can express. Never talk to another person about the resident in the resident's presence.

Adapted from Gwyther (1985).

Behavior problems are identified by the unit staff, and requests for consultations are submitted to the mental health coordinator. The coordinator then conducts an initial assessment of the resident to determine the urgency of the request and to identify which consultant should be called in on the case. Once all of the mental health professionals involved have completed their assessment, a mental health care plan is written in collaboration with the health care team on the resident's unit, and resident care conferences, which give the care team an opportunity to discuss the care planning process, are held. The coordinator initiates and coordinates the support functions provided by the other mental health professionals.

BEHAVIOR MANAGEMENT IN ACUTE CARE SETTINGS

Addressing behavior problems in the acute care setting requires a major shift in policy and attitude. Acute care facilities are geared toward rapid treatment of medical emergencies. The advent of DRGs has meant that patients undergoing elective procedures receive hospital care only during the most acute phase of their treatment. Acute care staff thus come to expect rapid turnover of their patient load and are trained to propel patients through laboratory work and diagnostic procedures rapidly. Members of the health care team tend to be highly skilled at identifying problems that are critical to a patient's physical progress and recovery, and less skilled in dealing with behavior problems. Such an environment is bound to aggravate a patient's tendency to experience behavior problems.

The unique needs of older adults are increasingly being recognized, and in the future, hospitals may establish geriatric care units staffed with professionals who understand the special needs of older adults. Currently, however, acute care settings are often inhospitable for older adults.

The most significant difference between acute care and long-term care is the length of stay. Turnover is rapid in acute care, with the average patient staying only a minimal number of days. Behavior problems often improve as adults adjust to their setting, but this may take as long as 6 months. Hence, some of the interventions that are appropriate for an older adult in a long-term care setting may not be appropriate in the acute care setting. Because of the very short period of time that patients remain in hospitals, the emphasis must be on interventions that can minimize stress in the short-run.

Reducing the Stress of Relocation

One cause of stress in acute care settings is repeated relocation of patients. In hospitals, patients are routinely moved from bed to bed, from room to room, and from unit to unit. The most difficult transition is the move from the operating room to the surgical recovery room. Having a family member sit with the patient may help orient and relax him or her, thus reducing the need for pain medication and/or physical restraint. Tests may also require frequent transport to and from other areas of the hospital.

Staff accustomed to such constant motion may fail to recognize that an older adult's capacity to adapt to rapid change is limited, and may cause confusion. To minimize the stress associated with relocation, hospital staff can take the following steps:

1. Provide all staff dealing with patients with inservice education about relocation stress.

2. Establish hospital-wide policies to reduce the amount of relocation of patients.

3. Try to have family members involved in the transporting of their family members.

4. Always explain to the patient and his or her family exactly what moves are to take place.

Older people often enjoy listening to music and may benefit from guided imagery, progressive relaxation, and other holistic health aides. Families should thus be encouraged to provide the patient with a radio with earphones and to provide a variety of relaxation tapes for use before and after a procedure.

Common Physical Causes of Behavior Problems

Staff also need to receive training on common immediate causes of behavior problems in older adults, including the following:

1. Infection, which can cause delirium. Even temperature elevations as slight as half a degree may indicate a serious infection that requires treatment

2. Medication, which frequently underlies behavior problems

3. Sensory deprivation, which may cause a noticeable decline in functioning by diminishing the patient's ability to perceive the environment

4. Stroke, which is frequently associated with verbally and physically aggressive behavior

Reducing Wandering in the Hospital

A form of problem behavior that is particularly common in acute care settings is wandering. To help prevent wandering by older patients, caregivers should:

1. Determine whether the patient wanders because of pain, hunger, thirst, or the need to use the bathroom, or because the patient is actually lost.

2. Try to keep the patient in the same room throughout his or her hospital stay.

3. Use familiar objects, such as pictures, to help the patient stay oriented.

4. Request a psychiatric consultation to determine whether a disturbance in the patient's sleep cycle may be responsible.

Caregivers should identify patients who wander and follow them when possible. They should also encourage families to stay with the patient during the night, or to hire a sitter to do so.

EVALUATION AND OUTCOMES

Success in managing behavior depends upon consistent follow-up. A follow-up system must be simple enough that it can be maintained over a long period of time. A short entry on the behavior management log (see Figure 14.1) enables staff to determine the effectiveness of a particular intervention at a glance. Detailed documentation belongs in the staff's progress note, not in the behavior management log. Ideally, the same person who deals with the requests for mental health consultations (i.e., the mental health coordinator) should be designated to document which interventions were tried and which were successful.

The first step in the process is to define the term improvement. To do so, it is essential that the evaluation form contain as detailed a description of the resident's behavior as possible. If the behavior cannot be eliminated, a change in its frequency or duration should be sought. It is also important to specify at what intervals the evaluator will check for improvement. Because residents deteriorate from day to day, improvement may not endure. If improvement is measured once over the course of a resident's stay in the facility, the interventions may reveal little effect. Frequent, intermittent evaluation will reveal progress more accurately. Assessment can be done weekly, monthly, or even as infrequently as once every 6 months.

The ultimate goal of behavior management is to improve the quality of a resident's life. Hence, even an improvement that lasts only a short period should be counted a success, as the following case study shows:

Mrs. Warren suffered from moderate to severe dementia, she moved little, and she did not eat. Her primary physician suggested a trial of

Ritalin. Within a week of receiving the medication, Mrs. Warren became more alert and resumed eating. Her daughter was thrilled. She was able to talk with her mother about some important issues, including Mrs. Warren's impending death. By the end of the month, Mrs. Warren suffered a second stroke and the Ritalin had to be discontinued. Although she never became alert to her surroundings, the intervention was documented a success.

Sometimes staff members' own anxiety fuels a resident's behavior problems. Staff may become so personally invested in making sure that the resident's evaluation demonstrates the treatment's success that they unintentionally barrage the resident with too many interventions. Although this flurry of activity may give the staff a sense that they are doing all they can, it may also stress the resident and even aggravate his or her behavior problems, as shown in the following case study:

Mr. Bennett, a 6-foot-tall resident, became emaciated. When his weight dropped below 100 pounds and he stopped walking, the staff became alarmed. The consulting psychiatrist diagnosed Mr. Bennett as having a schizoid personality disorder. The psychiatrist evaluated his medication and prescribed a new regime, changing both the dosage and the drug several times. The staff tried working with Mr. Bennett one on one, and the social worker called Mr. Bennett's daughter to come in to feed him. Although he improved slightly when his daughter began to visit more often, he remained essentially unchanged. When every possible medical intervention had been exhausted, the staff slowly ceased their efforts. Mr. Bennett's daughter objected to visiting so frequently and eventually developed her own physical problems. Mr. Bennett's condition worsened and the staff tried no further mental health interventions.

After one year, Mr. Bennett's condition remained unchanged. The flurry of interventions had ceased. He remained emaciated, but was not losing weight. Although he no longer walked, the staff described his condition as stable.

CONCLUSION

Behavior problems are best managed in an atmosphere of respect in which the uniqueness of all human beings is cherished. Such problems are best managed when the primary goal is not to control the behavior, but to understand it. The more caregivers are able to become students of behavior, the less inclined they will be to resort to the use of restraints.

REFERENCES

American Psychiatric Association. (1987). *Diagnostic and statistical manual of mental disorders* (DSM-III-R). Washington, DC. Author.

Burgio, L.D., Jones, L.T., Butler, F., & Engel, B.T. (1988). Behavior problems in an urban nursing home. *Journal of Gerontological Nursing, 14*(1), 31–34.

Burnside, I.M. (1980). *Psychosocial nursing care of the aged.* New York: McGraw-Hill.

Cohen-Mansfield, J. (1986). Agitated behaviors in the elderly. Preliminary results in the cognitively deteriorated. *Journal of the American Geriatrics Society, 34,* 722–727.

Combs, A., & Snygg, D. (1959). *Individualized behavior.* New York: Harper & Row.

Eaton, W.W., Reiger, D.A., Locke, B.Z., & Traube, C.A. (1981). The epidemiologic catchment area program of the National Institute of Mental Health. *Public Health Reports, 96,* 319–325.

Gwyther, L. (1985). *Care of Alzheimer' patients: A manual for nursing home staff* (pp. 92–93). Washington, DC: American Health Care Association and Alzheimer's Disease and Related Disorders Association.

Rovner, B.W., Kafonek, S., Filipp, L., Lucas, M.J., & Folstein, M.F. (1986). Prevalence of mental illness in a community nursing home. *American Journal of Psychiatry, 143*(11), 1446–1449.

Struble, L.M., & Sivertsen, L. (1987). Agitated behaviors in confused elderly patients. *Journal of Gerontological Nursing, 13*(11), 40–44.

Zimmer, J.G., Watson, N., & Treat, A. (1984). Behavioral problems among patients in skilled nursing facilities. *American Journal of Public Health, 74*(10), 1118–1120.

Part V

Legal, Regulatory, and Ethical Issues

Chapter 15

Legal and Regulatory Issues Governing the Use of Restraints

Proskauer Rose Goetz & Mendelsohn

Restraint use in long-term care facilities has become the subject of increasingly heated debate in the United States. The editorial columns of small-town newspapers and metropolitan tabloids, and even television news programs, denounce the practice as "punishment without crime." Several advocacy groups are mobilizing forces to increase public awareness of the prevalence of restraint use in long-term care facilities. The mounting social and media fervor surrounding the issue has even spilled over onto political ground. For example, the Omnibus Budget Reconciliation Act of 1987 (OBRA '87) contains language that significantly curtails the circumstances under which care providers may restrain residents and recognizes that residents have the right to be free from physical or chemical restraints. Likewise, many states have taken steps aimed at curbing the use of restraints through civil, and sometimes criminal, sanctions.

Some long-term care providers are troubled by the recent anti-restraint movement and have voiced concerns that the lack of availability of restraints may aggravate already crisis-level staffing shortages, lead to injuries to residents, and increase providers' potential liability for such injuries.

Proskauer has prepared this chapter to provide an accurate explanation of the legal and regulatory issues governing the use of restraints. This information is made available with the understanding that it is general in nature and is not intended as legal or professional advice with respect to the specific circumstances of any particular health care provider. Therefore, before any action is taken based upon the information contained herein, the reader should consult with professional advisors on the specific actions considered. For further information on legal and regulatory issues, contact Malcolm J. Harkins, III, or Pamela Beth Small at (202) 416–6800.

This chapter examines the practices, devices, and forms of treatment that constitute physical and chemical restraints and describes the circumstances under which these restraints may be used under the OBRA '87 guidelines. It also analyzes the circumstances under which liability has been imposed on providers for the nonuse and misuse of restraints and describes how potential liability is altered by new and more stringent federal and state legislation and regulations governing restraint use. The chapter concludes with suggested strategies that health care providers may implement in order to reduce their exposure.

DEFINITION OF RESTRAINTS

Federal Definition

Under federal law, restraints are considered to be any safety device, appliance, or medication that is imposed for the purpose of discipline or convenience and is not required to treat a medical symptom. Restraints generally are divided into two types: physical and chemical. The Health Care Financing Administration's (HCFA) *Interpretive Guidelines* to OBRA '87 define physical restraints as:

> Any manual method or physical or mechanical device, material, or equipment attached or adjacent to the resident's body that the individual cannot remove easily which restricts free movement or normal access to one's body.
>
> Physical restraints include leg restraints, arm restraints, hand mitts, soft ties or vests, and wheelchair safety bars. (HCFA, 1992, p. P-76)

The *Interpretive Guidelines* define a chemical restraint as "a psychopharmacologic drug used for discipline or convenience and not required to treat medical symptoms" (HCFA, p. P-76). According to the *Guidelines*, "discipline" refers to actions taken for the purpose of punishing or penalizing a resident; "convenience" refers to actions taken "to control resident behavior or maintain residents with a lesser amount of effort by the facility and not in the resident's best interests (HCFA, p. P-76). Under OBRA '87, any type of drug, including antihistamines or other hypnotics, although generally considered relatively benign, is now considered a "chemical restraint" unless it is administered pursuant to a physician's order for a specified medical condition in a specified dose.

State Definitions

Most state definitions of restraints employ a "subjective use" analysis. Under such an analysis, whether or not a device or medication is deemed a restraint depends on the purpose for which it is used. The OBRA '87 *Guidelines* effectively abolished this "subjective use" analysis for physical and chemical restraints by keying restraint use to whether the restraint is imposed for discipline or convenience and not for a particular medical symptom. An example of a state "subjective use" test is the Supreme Court of Wisconsin decision in *Kujawski v. Arbor View Health Care Center* 139 Wisc.2d 455, 407 N.W.2d (1987), in which the court, relying on the state "subjective use" definition of physical restraints, found that a wheelchair safety belt was not a restraint because the belt was used to keep the resident from falling out of the wheelchair, rather than to modify behavior. The *Guidelines* make it clear, however, that the OBRA '87 definition would not support such a conclusion.

PREVALENCE OF RESTRAINTS

Restraint use in long-term care facilities is pervasive. The vast majority of such facilities use restraints (Farnsworth, 1973), and various studies report that 25%–84.6% of residents in skilled nursing facilities have restraint orders (Evans & Strumpf, 1989). According to federal surveys in 1989, about 41% of all long-term care facility residents were placed in restraints in 1989 (New York Times, 1991). Federal survey data compiled in November, 1992, indicate national average percentages of 22% for physically restrained and 27% for chemically restrained nursing home residents.

RATIONALES FOR RESTRAINT USE

The most common rationale for restraint use is the protection of the resident or others from harm (Frengley & Mion, 1986). Other rationales include the reduction in nursing time required to monitor restrained residents, and concern about the facility's legal liability for failure to restrain residents who injure themselves or others.

Protection of the Resident and Others

No scientific basis supports the conclusion that restraints help to safeguard residents from injury (Rubenstein, Miller, Postel, & Evans, 1983). To the contrary, a substantial volume of scientific research suggests that restraints can reduce a resident's functional capacity and create problems with elimination and conditions such as aspiration pneumonia, circulatory obstruction, cardiac stress, skin abrasions or breakdown, poor appetite and dehydration, and accidental death by strangulation. Furthermore, restraint use has been linked with abnormal changes in body chemistry, basal metabolic rate, and blood volume; low blood pressure upon standing; contractures, edema of the lower extremities, and pressure sores; decreased muscle mass and muscle tone/strength; bone demineralization; overgrowth of opportunistic organisms; and changes in electroencephalograms (Evans & Strumpf, 1989).

Reduction in Staffing Requirements

Restraint use does not appear to relieve staffing problems. Restrained residents generally must be released for at least 10 minutes in every 2-hour period during normal waking hours to allow for repositioning and exercise. Many commentators have argued that, given this requirement, providers cannot comply fully with restraint release regulations and maintain the reimbursed nursing ratio. One study, by the Kendal Corporation, suggested that to release and care for a restrained resident properly requires 4.58 hours per patient per day, which is well in excess of the reimbursed ratio of any state. Furthermore, many facilities that have limited or eliminated restraint use have reported that employee morale increases and turnover decreases, and that residents are far more manageable and need less supervision without restraints (Evans & Strumpf, 1989).Hence, it appears that, contrary to popular belief, restraining residents may have a detrimental effect on minimum staffing requirements in long-term care facilities.

Legal Ramifications of the Nonuse of Restraints

Few precedents support successful malpractice claims against long-term care facilities based upon a failure to restrain. In fact, no reported case has yet been successful against a facility solely for failure to restrain a resident. Indeed, restraint misuse has provoked far more litigation than has nonuse.

There are several reasons for the dearth of cases that hold providers liable for injuries that result from the failure to restrain a resident. First, there is little economic incentive to pursue such a claim, because the amount of obtainable damages is very low as a result of the limited earning potential and lifespan of an older adult. Second, it is difficult to establish a causal connection between the failure to restrain and the injury. Third, courts have proved reluctant to expand the general standard of care that long-term care facilities owe residents to include a duty to restrain.

PROVIDER LIABILITY FOR
MISUSE OR NONUSE OF RESTRAINTS

Standards of Care for the Use of Restraints

Common Law Standard Most jurisdictions follow the traditional common law nursing home standard of care that, while recognizing that "[a] nursing home is not the insurer of the safety of its patients" (*Nichols v. Green Acres Rest Home, Inc.*, 1971)[1], requires such facilities to use a reasonable level of care to protect residents from any injury that might reasonably be anticipated (*Bezark v. Kostner Manor, Inc.*, 1961).[2] The majority view of the standard of care that a facility owes to a resident is based on the resident's physical and mental condition.[3]

Statutory and Regulatory Standard Several states have established the standard of care that providers owe care facility residents by requiring that facilities include statutory standards in their contracts with incoming residents (*Stiffelman v. Abrams*, 1983). Indeed, reliance on statutory and regulatory standards of care seems to be a growing trend, under which a deviation from a restraint-related statute or regulation is considered prima facie evidence of negligence.

The Missouri Supreme Court has held that a cause of action can be maintained based on the Missouri "Residents' Bill of Rights,"

---

[1]See also *Bezark v. Kostner Manor, Inc.*, 172 N.E.2d 424, 426 (Ill. App. Ct. 1961); *Juhnke v. Evangelical Lutheran Good Samaritan Society*, 634 P.2d 1132, 1136 (Kan. Ct. App. 1981); *McGillivray v. Rapides Iberia Management Enterprises*, 493 So.2d 819, 821-22 (La. Ct. App. 1986); *Oswald v. Rapides Iberia Management Enterprises*, 452 So. 2d 1258, 1262 (La. Ct. App. 1984); *Collier v. Ami, Inc.*, 254 So.2d 170, 173-74 (La. Ct. App. 1971). A Texas court has recognized that it "is the duty of a hospital to provide for the care and protection of its patients, and in the exercise of this duty the hospital is required to provide such reasonable care as the patient's known condition requires." See *Golden Villa Nursing Home, Inc. v. Smith*, 674 S.W.2d 343, 348 (Tex.Ct. App. 1984).

[2]The court in *Bezark* also noted that "as to dangers reasonably to be anticipated from acts of other persons under the hospitals' control, reasonable care and attention must be exercised for the safety and well being of their patients, in proportion to the circumstances and their ability to look after their own safety." With regard to the condition of the premises, see *Facey v. Merkle*, 148 A.2d 261, 264 (Conn. 1959).

[3]A few states have sought to impose an extraordinarily high standard of care on long-term care facilities. A recent decision by the Indiana Supreme Court, for instance, expanded the so-called "common carrier exception" to include long-term care facilities. This exception is normally reserved for airlines, ships, trains, and other modes of transportation in which people voluntarily relinquish control over their persons and place their safety in the hands of others. This decision rests on untested and dubious legal underpinnings, and should be viewed as an aberration from the majority "reasonable care" standard. See *Stropes v. Heritage House Children's Center of Shelbyville, Inc. and Robert Griffin*, 547 N.E.2d 244 (Ind. 1989).

which requires that each resident be "free from mental and physical abuse, and free from chemical and physical restraints . . ."(Mo. Ann. Stat. §199.088, 1983). The court reasoned that the purpose of the Residents' Bill of Rights was to "protect the health and safety of citizens who are unable fully to take care of themselves, particularly the more elderly persons . . ." (*Stiffelman v. Abrams*, 1983).

Similarly, California law has held that long-term care facility residents have a statutory private right of action for any violation of residents' rights, including the right to be free from restraints (*California Administrative Code* title 22 §72527(a)(8), 1990; *West's Annotated California Code*—Health & Safety §1430(b), 1990).

Thus, the standard of care that providers owe long-term care facility residents has been defined by the statutes and regulations governing that care. Evidence of the standard of care has also been found in the policies and procedures adopted by long-term care facilities.

Provider Liability for Nonuse of Restraints

Harm to the Resident   Every reported case in which a provider has been held liable for a restraint-related incident has required proof of some type of separate negligence, such as improper assessment of the resident, failure to monitor him or her, or failure to respond to an accident in a timely and professional manner. Almost every case in which providers have been held liable for the nonuse of restraints resulting in harm to the resident has involved the failure to provide adequate supervision for residents who wander. The following are some examples:

1. In *Booty v. Kentwood Manor Nursing Home, Inc.* (1985), the court found a care facility liable for failure to supervise a resident who wandered out of the facility and fell, ultimately dying from injuries sustained in the fall. The court based its decision on the finding that although the facility had responded reasonably to the problem of wandering by installing an alarm system on exit doors, these doors had been propped open solely for the convenience of the facility's staff, thus allowing the resident to leave the building unnoticed.

2. In *Fields v. Senior Citizens Center, Inc. of Coushatta* (1988), the court found a care facility liable for the death of a 68-year-old resident who wandered out of the facility onto a nearby road and was struck by a van driven by the resident's daughter. The court found that although the facility had a door alarm system installed, the system was disengaged at the time the resident left

the facility because staff found the alarm annoying. Further, the court found that nursing stations were left vacant, thus contributing to the lack of supervision at the facility.

3. In *Golden Villa Nursing, Inc. v. Smith* (1984), a resident was left unsupervised for about an hour and was last seen on the back porch of the facility. The resident wandered onto an adjacent highway and was hit by a motorcycle. The Texas Court of Appeals held that the facility's prior knowledge of the resident's tendency to wander toward the highway placed the defendants under a duty to "take such tendencies into consideration in protecting and providing for her" and to provide reasonable care in accordance with the known mental and physical conditions of the resident. The court also noted that a mere showing "of conformity with industry supervisory standards does not preclude a showing of negligence and of breach of duty in specific situations."

4. A departure from the prevailing trend is *Kujawski v. Arbor View Health Care Center* (1987), in which the Wisconsin Supreme Court held that the jury could determine without expert testimony whether restraints should have been used. The case was sent back for a new trial, but it was subsequently settled.

5. In *McGillivray v. Rapides Iberia Management Enterprises* (1986), the court held a care facility liable for failure to monitor or supervise a resident who was known to wander and for whom his children and his physician had authorized physical restraints when necessary to protect against his tendency to wander.

A common theme in each of these cases is the courts' unwillingness to hold that care providers have a duty to restrain. Rather, courts emphasize the providers' duty to supervise and provide reasonable care. As one court noted, "The findings . . . refer not to the failure of nurses to place Mr. Fox in the harness that night, but to their failure to guard against his leaving the premises" (*McGillivray v. Rapides Iberia Management Enterprises*, 1986).

Harm to Other Residents   There are no reported cases of providers being held liable for any harm that one resident may have inflicted upon another based specifically on a "failure to restrain" theory. However, in *Juhnke v. Evangelical Lutheran Good Samaritan Society* (1981), the court found that a care facility breached its duty to provide reasonable care for a resident who was struck by another resident based upon proof that the resident who struck the plaintiff had a well-known tendency to be "very belligerent [and to] wander around the nursing home and in the rooms of other patients, pushing, tripping and hurting others." Although the court in that case did not base its decision on a failure to restrain the aggressive resident, the court did recognize the principle that "one who takes charge of a third person whom he knows or should know to be likely to cause bodily harm to another if not controlled is under a duty to exercise reasonable care to control the third person to prevent him from doing such harm" (*Juhnke v. Evangelical Lutheran Good Samaritan Society*, 1981).[4] As these cases illustrate, providers' liability for injuries sustained by a resident as a result of another resident's aggressive behavior has not been defined by whether or not the aggressive resident should have been restrained. Rather, it is derived from a larger duty to take "reasonable care" to protect residents from known dangers.

Provider Liability for Misuse of Restraints

Failure to use restraints properly and to supervise restrained residents has increased providers' legal exposure far more than has the nonuse of restraints. Research reveals at least 40 recent instances in which residents strangled as a result of improperly used safety vests alone. One such death resulted in a $39.4 million jury award to the family of an 84-year-old woman who strangled in a vest in a Houston care facility (Green & Pollack, 1990).[5]

Providers have been held liable for the misuse of restraints in the following cases:

1. In *Cramer v. Theda Clark Memorial Hospital* 172 N.W.2d 427 (Wisc. 1970), a nurse brought a supper tray to a resident who was restrained and untied one of the restraints so that the resident could eat. The nurse then left the room without retying the restraint. The resident untied the other restraint, and while attempting to stand, fell and fractured his hip. The court held the hospital liable, largely because of its failure to abide by its own policy and procedure for monitoring residents.

2. In *Dusine v. Golden Shores Convalescent Center, Inc.* 249 So.2d. 40 (Fla. Dist. Ct. App. 1971), a resident was injured when left unattended in a vest restraint. Liability hinged on a lack of supervision rather than misuse of a restraint, since state regulations required extensive supervision of restrained residents.

---

[4]See also *Rosemont, Inc. v. Marshall* 481 So.2d 1126 (Ala. 1985), and *Bezark v. Kostner Manor, Inc.* 29 Ill. App.2d 106, 172 N.E.2d 424 (Ill. App. Ct. 1961).

[5]Counsel for the defendants in this case have indicated that they will seek to overturn the award as excessive.

3. In *Fleming v. Prince George's County* 277 Md. 685, 358 A.2d 892 (1976), an older patient, driven by a "psychotic" desire induced by Librium and Valium ordered by her physician as restraints, attempted to escape and fell seven floors.

4. In *Dow v. State* 50 N.Y.S.2d 342, 183 Misc. 674 (1944), a hospital was found liable for applying an inadequate restraint and failing to supervise a "manic-depressive" patient.

5. In *Horton v. Niagara Falls Memorial Medical Center* 380 N.Y.S.2d 116, 51 A.D.2d 152 (1976), a New York court found a hospital liable for failing to supervise a patient restrained with a posey vest and wristlets who fell out of a second story window.

6. In *Morningside Hospital & Training School for Nurses v. Pennington* 189 Okla. 170, 114 P.2d 943 (1941), a hospital was found negligent for failure to supervise an improperly restrained patient.

7. In *Northrup v. Archbishop Bergan Mercy Hospital* 575 F.2d 605 (8th Cir. 1978), a hospital was held liable for the use of a restraint from which the patient was known to be able to escape and for failure to supervise the restrained patient.

As with the "failure to restrain" cases, courts that impose liability for the misuse of restraints tend to focus on the adequacy of supervision. One theme common to these cases is that once a facility restrains a resident, it bears greater responsibility for supervising the resident and for ensuring that the restraint does not harm the resident.

FEDERAL AND STATE EFFORTS TO LIMIT RESTRAINT USE

The Omnibus Budget Reconciliation Act of 1987 (OBRA '87)

OBRA '87 contains specific provisions that outline the circumstances under which restraints may be used in long-term care facilities. Implemented in 1991, the restraint provision states that each resident has the "right to be free from physical or mental abuse, corporal punishment, involuntary seclusion, and any physical or chemical restraints imposed for purposes of discipline or convenience and not required to treat the resident's medical symptoms" (OBRA, 1987).

The term *chemical restraint* was excised from the text of the final rules, in recognition of the fact that many drugs are designed to restrain certain behaviors. Drugs become "chemical restraints" only when used without proper indications, in excessive doses, or for excessive periods of time. Hence, the final rule provides that "the resident has the right to be free from any physical restraints imposed or psychoactive drug administered for purposes of discipline or convenience, and not required to treat the resident's medical symptoms" (42 Fed. Reg. §483.13(a), 1991).[6]

The OBRA '87 provisions further state that:

> Restraints may only be imposed to ensure the physical safety of the resident or other residents, and only upon the written order of a physician that specifies the duration and the circumstances under which the restraints are to be used (except in emergency circumstances specified by the Secretary) until such an order could reasonably be obtained. (OBRA, 1987)

Physical Restraints　The OBRA '87 restraint provisions represent a significant departure from previous state-level attempts to regulate restraint use. These provisions eliminate the distinction between physical restraints and devices used to position a resident (postural supports) or safety devices. This is in contrast to state regulations that generally distinguish between physical restraints used to control or modify a resident's behavior and postural supports designed to achieve proper body alignment or to prevent falls.

The HCFA *Interpretive Guidelines* to OBRA '87 clarify and expand upon the OBRA '87 restraint provisions, declaring that:

> *Discipline* is any action taken by the facility for the purpose of punishing or penalizing residents.
> *Convenience* is any action taken by the facility to control resident behavior or maintain residents with a lesser amount of effort by the facility and not in the residents' best interest. . . .
> If the resident needs emergency care, restraints may be used for brief periods to permit medical treatment to proceed unless the facility has noticed that the resident has previously made a valid refusal of the treatment in question. (HCFA, 1992, p. P-77)

The restraint regulations are merely one method of achieving OBRA '87's overall goal of improving quality of care and quality of life for long-term care residents. Medicare and Medicaid requirements for long-term care facilities under OBRA '87 envision consis-

---

[6]A proposed rule issued for comment proposes a return to the use of the term "chemical restraints." See 57 Fed. Reg. 4516, 4517, 4530-31 (Feb. 5, 1992). These rules, if finalized in substantially the same form as proposed, would significantly change the federal restraint standard by codifying not only a definition of physical and chemical restraint, but also by specifying when a long-term care facility may use physical and chemical restraints, how those restraints are to be applied, and what documentation will be required. See 57 Fed. Reg. 4516,4517-20, 4530-31 (Feb. 5, 1992). As of April 22, 1992, the HCFA acknowledged receiving more than a thousand sets of comments on these proposed rules and predicted that it would need a significant amount of time to analyze the comments and then amend and reissue the rule.

tent requirements for care facilities. The regulations focus on actual facility performance in meeting residents' needs; accordingly, enforcement of the regulations is undertaken from the perspective of quality of care and quality of life for long-term care residents.

The regulations state that residents have the right to self-determination and participation (42 Fed. Reg. §483.15(b), 1991), and mandate that residents receive "the necessary care and services to attain or maintain the highest practicable physical, mental, and psychosocial well-being, in accordance with the comprehensive assessment and plan of care" (42 Fed. Reg. §483.25, 1991). Thus, the perceived goals for the care of older adults are shifting from the earlier concept of facility compliance with health regulations to the more recent one of a facility's active promotion of the health and well-being of older adults in long-term care settings.

As mentioned previously, restraints contribute demonstrably to residents' ill health in a variety of ways (Evans & Strumpf, 1989). Prolonged immobility resulting from restraint use has been shown to produce negative outcomes to patients' skin, such as bruises, cuts, and pressure sores; to decrease residents' musculoskeletal function by causing wasting of muscles, contractures of the extremities, and increased fractures resulting from bone loss; and to cause other negative physiological and psychological effects (Evans & Strumpf, 1989).

The focus on quality of care and quality of life emphasizes the provider's duty to care for residents proactively so that at the very least, a resident's condition does not deteriorate, and at the most, a resident who has no specific health problems upon admission to the facility does not subsequently develop problems as a result of conditions in the facility. Hence, the new restraint regulations must be read in conjunction with the other quality of care and quality of life provisions.

For example, if a resident has no pressure sores upon entering a facility, the facility must take active steps to prevent the development of sores. If sores do develop, the facility must be able to show that the sores developed as a result of an unavoidable clinical condition (42 Fed. Reg. §483.25(c)(1), 1991). Residents who have a normal range of motion when they enter the facility must not be allowed to experience a reduction in their range of motion, "unless the resident's clinical condition demonstrates that a reduction in range of motion is unavoidable" (42 Fed. Reg. §483.25(e)(1), 1991). Residents who have a limited range of motion must receive nursing services that increase their range of motion and/or prevent further decrease in their range of motion (42 Fed. Reg. §483.25(e)(2), 1991). Hence, a provider must be aware that restraining a resident improperly may, in itself, constitute a violation; however, even proper restraint use may produce conditions in residents that violate the quality of care and quality of life regulations.

Use of Drugs as Restraints A 1989 survey of long-term care facilities revealed that 50% of the residents received some type of psychotropic medication (Nursing Home Community Coalition of New York State, 1989). Similarly, a Harvard Medical School survey of 55 long-term care facilities found that 55% of the residents received at least one psychoactive medication. Antipsychotic medications were administered to 39%, of whom 18% received two or more such drugs, which can create dangerous risks if administered in error (Avorn, Dreyer, Connelly, & Soumerai, 1989).

A Harvard Medical School study of the use of psychoactive medications with intermediate-care facility residents contained other startling statistics. Data on prescriptions and actual use of medications were recorded for 1 month for 850 patients in 12 intermediate-care facilities in Massachusetts. Among the residents studied, 58% received psychoactive medication and 26% received antipsychotic medication (Beers, Avorn, Soumerai, Everitt, Sherman, & Salem, 1988). Similar pictures have emerged from the National Nursing Home Study Pretest and from Medicaid records in Illinois (Beers et al., 1988).

These studies reveal a practice of drug use with older adults that borders on the indiscriminate. The goal of OBRA '87 is to eliminate such indiscriminate drug use (42 Fed. Reg. §483.25(l), 1991). For example, a resident who has not used antipsychotic drugs previously may be given them only to treat a specific condition; and residents who currently use antipsychotic drugs must receive gradual dose reductions or behavioral interventions unless these measures are clinically contradicted. The regulations contemplate that residents will be drug free unless drugs are necessary, properly prescribed, and properly administered (42 Fed. Reg. §483.15(l), (m), 1991).

Far from being an isolated set of new requirements for long-term care, the OBRA '87 restraint regulations comprise one of many aspects of the regulatory resident care regime. Limiting unnecessary restraint and drug use is now integral to improved care.

Mandatory Less Restrictive Solutions

The use of solutions that are less restrictive than restraints is mandatory under the new resident care regime. Measures that are classified as less restrictive may include pillows, wedge cushions, pads, removable lap trays, and exercise as a means to provide better postural support, to achieve proper body alignment, and to prevent contractures. Moreover, the facility must have documented evidence of consultation with an occupational or physical therapist regarding the use of less restrictive supportive devices before resorting to physical restraints (HCFA, 1992).

After a trial of less restrictive measures, the facility may decide that a restraint would "promote the care and services necessary for the resident to attain or maintain the highest practicable wellbeing" (HCFA, 1992, p. P-76). In such instances, the use of the restraining device first must be explained to the resident, a family member, or a legal representative. If the resident, family member, or legal representative agrees to this treatment alternative, then the restraining device may be used for a specific period of time during which the restraint will enhance the resident's independence.

The HCFA *Guidelines'* brief treatment of the need to consult with the resident, family member, or legal representative belies the complicated legal issues that may arise. For example, OBRA '87 gives residents the right to refuse treatment (*Federal Register*, vol. 54, p. 5360, 1989; 42 Fed. Reg. §483.10(b)(4), 1991). Hence, a resident who constantly removes a catheter or nasogastric tube may not be restrained to prevent such behavior—the resident is refusing treatment. According to HCFA, refusal of treatment must be "persistent and continuously documented" (*Federal Register*, vol. 54, p. 5321, 1989).

When a resident refuses restraint use, federal law provides that "unless [the resident is] adjudged incompetent or otherwise found to be incapacitated under the laws of the State, [he or she has the right to] participate in planning care and treatment or changes in care and treatment" (42 Fed. Reg. §483.10(d)(3), 1991). Hence, residents must be allowed to participate in treatment decisions, and residents may refuse restraints. It is surprising, considering the source, that the federal regulations suggest that if a resident refuses restraints and yet might endanger others if not restrained, the facility should discharge the resident on the grounds that it is unable to provide proper treatment (*Federal Register*, vol. 54, p. 5321, 1989). Therefore, if a legally competent resident refuses restraints and the care facility adjudges itself incapable of providing the treatment that the resident needs, discharge is an option.

If the resident is not considered capable of making treatment decisions, the provider then must ask family members (who may disagree among themselves) or a legal representative (if one is available) to decide. However, state law may restrict the use of surrogates for decision making. The law of the District of Columbia, for example, presumes that the resident is capable of deciding about treatment, and this presumption can be rebutted only by a medical certification; surrogate decision-making is illegal if the person has a relative or a power of attorney vested in another individual.

VALID RESTRAINT USE

Under current law, residents of long-term care facilities must be free from physical restraints and psychoactive drugs *unless* the restraints are authorized by a physician, in writing, for a specified period of time, or unless they are used in an emergency.

HCFA's *Guidelines* provide a single exception to the procedures for using restraints: such restraints can be administered without a written order from a physician when life-threatening medical symptoms, such as dehydration, electrolyte imbalance, and urinary blockage, are present. In such cases, a restraint may be used temporarily to provide necessary lifesaving treatment. In an emergency, however, a professional staff member, identified in the facility's policy and procedures manual as having the power to authorize emergency restraint use, should authorize the restraint use. In addition, that professional staff member must report the restraint use to the resident's physician promptly.

The *Guidelines* treat wheelchair safety bars, geri-chairs, and hand mitts applied to keep the resident from removing a nasogastric tube as restraints, overturning the once-accepted safety justification for restrictions on a resident's movement. Also, although bedrails are not considered a restraint, to the extent that they keep a resident from leaving a bed voluntarily they are considered an "accident hazard" under the new regulations (42 Fed. Reg. §483.25(h)(l), 1991). The *Guidelines* define *accident hazards* as "physical features in the nursing facility environment that can endanger a resident's safety" (HCFA, 1987, p. P-97). Hence, facilities that are accustomed to the use of bedrails as a standard feature must be aware that rails are no longer considered justifiable as safety devices.[7]

With respect to drug use, the Guidelines endorse strict adherence to prescribed amounts as well as documentation of prescribed and actual use. Facilities must be prepared to comply with the strict documentation and use requirements for psychoactive drugs.

---

[7]This may put providers in an untenable position; for example, under Minnesota law, bedrails must be used for every resident.

ENFORCEMENT: INTERMEDIATE SANCTIONS UNDER OBRA '87

Termination of a facility's certification and transfer of its residents are penalties for noncompliance under OBRA '87. However, since these measures have a negative effect on resident care, termination and transfer are the ultimate penalties—employed as a last resort against providers whose facilities are out of compliance. Therefore, OBRA '87 mandates that state authorities put into effect "intermediate sanctions," in the form of denial of payment, civil monetary penalties, and temporary management for deficient facilities (42 U.S.C.A. §1396r(h)(1)(B)[1992]). States must impose civil monetary penalties for each day during which the facility is out of compliance.

Currently, complete federal rules for intermediate sanctions have not been implemented; however, states were required to implement intermediate sanctions by October 1, 1989 (42 U.S.C.A. §1396r(h)(2)(B)(i)[1992]). The responsibility to do so rests on the states because, under federal statutes, federal authorities will deny federal financial participation, also known as FFP, to states that have noncompliant facilities (42 U.S.C.A. §1396r(h)(3) (C)(i)[1992]). Since that time, various states have proposed and implemented civil money penalties amounting to thousands of dollars per day, triggered, for example, by a pattern of either serious or life-threatening deficiencies within a facility (*Annotated Code of Maryland*, Health—General, §19-1405, 1990 & Supp. 1992).

A "serious" condition, under some state laws, is defined not as a life-threatening health or fire safety condition, but as one that violates departmental regulations and is likely to endanger the life, safety, or health of residents. Hence, it is conceivable that widespread, improperly authorized restraint use could lead to a deficiency citation and civil money penalties.

In cases of noncompliance, federal authorities may also impose additional civil monetary penalties upon providers, not to exceed $10,000, and install temporary management (42 U.S.C.A. §1396r(h)(3)(C)(ii)[1992]). Exclusion from Medicare is also possible (42 U.S.C.A. §1320a-7a[1992]). Because the state and federal sanctions are parallel and concurrent, the financial liability for providers is potentially significant.

State Level Restraint Limitations

State and Regulatory Restraint Limitations Under the laws of various states, the right to be free from restraints is an element of each state's Residents' Bill of Rights. The definitions of physical restraints typically are similar to those stated by federal law. In addition, most states also provide for the humane use of restraints and contain further limitations. Mechanical supports usually are designated specifically as distinct from restraints. However, whether this distinction will continue to be accepted remains to be seen.

Criminal Sanctions In some states, restraint misuse is considered a form of elder abuse, which can have regulatory, civil, and possibly criminal ramifications. Under California law, for example, "physical abuse" of older adults is defined as including the "use of a physical or chemical restraint, medication, or isolation without authorization, or for a purpose other than for which it was ordered, including, but not limited to, for staff convenience, for punishment, or for a period beyond that for which it was ordered" (Cal. [Welfare and Institutions] Code §15610(c)(6) & 15632[1900]). Thus, misuse of restraints is classified as elder abuse.

California law further provides that:

> Any person who fails to report an instance of elder or dependent adult abuse which he or she *knows to exist or reasonably should know to exist* . . . is guilty of a misdemeanor and shall be punished by imprisonment in the county jail not exceeding six months, by a fine of not exceeding $1,000.00 or by both that fine and imprisonment. (Cal.[Welfare and Institutions] Code §15634(d)[1990]; emphasis added)

Essentially, this provision criminalizes negligent failure to report restraint misuse.

Providers should be aware that failure to report an instance of restraint misuse thus is criminally punishable. The provider's duty is double: not only must restraints be used carefully within the confines of the law, but any departure from the legal restrictions must be reported, in order to avoid possible criminal sanctions.

Under New York law, "mistreatment" is defined as "inappropriate use of medications, inappropriate isolation or inappropriate use of physical or chemical restraints on or of a patient or resident of a residential health care facility . . ." (New York Consolidated Law Service, Public Health §12(1), 1989). The regulations state that penalties accrue to both the abuser and any person who fails to report such abuse (New York Consolidated Law Service, Public Health §12-b, 1989).

Penalties include a fine of up to $1,000. If the violation of any health provision is willful, it is a misdemeanor, and punishable by up to 1 year in prison, a fine of up to $2,000, or both. This law applies to instances of willful mistreatment or other willful violations that are not otherwise categorized as a crime (New York Consolidated Law Service, Public Health §12b(2), 1989). One nurse who physically restrained a resident against his will has been convicted under this statute (*People v. Coe*, 1988).

Under Rhode Island law, "mistreatment" is defined as:

[I]nappropriate use of medications, isolation, or use of physical or chemical restraints as punishment, for staff convenience, as a substitute for treatment or care, in conflict with a physician's order, or in quantities which inhibit effective care or treatment, which harms or is likely to harm the resident. (*General Laws of Rhode Island* §23-17.8-1(b)[1900])

This statute is subject to broad interpretation, because if a restraint is used in a way that is *likely to harm* but that does not actually harm the resident, a penalty may still apply. Yet, even with proper use of any type of restraint, whether physical or chemical, the possibility of harm to a resident is likely.

Rhode Island law, like California law, imposes an affirmative duty to report mistreatment together with the risk of incurring a misdemeanor and a fine; anyone who induces another to fail to report, or who fails to report, an incident of mistreatment is guilty of a misdemeanor and subject to a fine (*General Laws of Rhode Island*, §23-17.8-3(A), (B), (C)[1900]). "Knowing" violations of these provisions can result in imprisonment for 3 years and fines of up to $3,000.

In summary, state standards that specify the intent required with respect to potentially criminally sanctioned restraint use vary in their wording from "aware or should have been aware," to "knowing," to "willful"—creating wide opportunity for Medicaid fraud control units, survey agencies, and prosecutors to penalize facilities that use restraints. Ironically, the increase in civil and criminal penalties coincides with a severe nationwide nursing shortage.

Private Causes of Action OBRA '87 and the growing social and medical movement to limit restraint use may alter the potential liability for nonuse and misuse of restraints dramatically. As discussed below, OBRA '87 and the corresponding change in the medical position regarding the appropriateness of using restraints may alter the standard of care analysis, making it less likely that a facility will incur liability for failing to restrain, but more likely that facilities will be exposed to liability for misusing.

Nonuse of Restraints: Harm to Self Courts have displayed great reluctance to recognize any duty to restrain residents. The OBRA '87 changes and growing medical concern over restraint use make it likely that no such duty will be recognized. Cases that impose liability on facilities focus on adequacy of supervision and monitoring, not on whether a facility had a duty to restrain a resident. The

OBRA '87 changes and the restraint minimization movement are clear indicators that the courts' focus will remain on whether facilities have monitored and supervised residents adequately, not on whether facilities should have restrained a resident. Furthermore, OBRA '87 provides a limited exception that allows restraints to be used if they are necessary to prevent harm to the resident, provided that a physician's order specifies the circumstances under which restraints are to be used and the duration of their uses. Thus, although the use of restraints in such limited circumstances must be prescribed specifically, and the restraint order documented and complied with meticulously, facilities may still restrain a resident if the resident's behavior poses a danger to him or herself that can be alleviated by restraint use.

Nonuse of Restraints: Harm to Others   The failure to use restraints to protect residents from other residents is a far more problematic concept than is the failure to restrain to prevent harm to the restrained resident. Few reported cases impose liability on a facility for injuries that a resident has sustained as a result of another resident's aggressive behavior, and no reported case imposes liability on a facility based on a "failure to restrain" theory.

Some commentators have argued that the OBRA '87 changes present providers with a dilemma: restrain an aggressive resident and risk regulatory and legal liability for misuse of restraints, or refrain from restraining and risk liability based on a failure to provide for the safety of the harmed resident. However, OBRA '87 does permit the use of restraints to protect other residents from harm, provided that the facility restrains only under a physician's order that specifies the duration of use and circumstances under which restraints may be used, except in emergency situations until such an order reasonably can be obtained. Thus, OBRA '87 does not prevent long-term care facilities from restraining aggressive residents. Facilities may restrain aggressive residents, but only under limited circumstances and under a highly specific physician's order ("as needed" orders for restraint use are unacceptable under OBRA '87).

Misuse of Restraints   Misuse of restraints accounts for the majority of cases that involve provider liability for restraint-related claims. The OBRA '87 changes make it likely that this trend will continue, if not intensify. As mentioned earlier, a growing number of states are looking to statutory and regulatory definitions to determine the standard of care that providers owe care facility residents. To the extent that OBRA '87 imposes strict limitations on restraint use, the failure to adhere strictly to these requirements may be considered prima facie evidence of negligence. Under such a theory, suits could take a variety of forms, ranging from wrongful death to false imprisonment.

Currently, there are few reported cases of facilities that have incurred liability for the misuse of restraints. However, the stricter requirements of OBRA '87 and the correspondingly more stringent standard of care associated with restraint use increase the likelihood that more instances of the misuse of restraints will be reported and acted upon by residents, their relatives, and regulators.

STRATEGIES FOR COMPLIANCE

Familiarity with the *Interpretive Guidelines for Surveyors*

Before the implementation of OBRA '87 in 1991, regulations governing restraint use in long-term care facilities substantially exposed facilities to regulatory deficiency citations. In 1989, one in five facilities in the nation was cited for restraint violations during federal certification surveys. Under OBRA '87, this exposure will increase dramatically. Hence, it is important that administrators and directors of nursing be knowledgeable about the more stringent OBRA '87 requirements.

Familiarity with the HCFA *Guidelines* is essential to provide administrators and directors of nursing with insight into the surveyors' perspective when reviewing a facility for compliance with the restraint regulations. Although the *Guidelines* themselves are by no means the final word on how to comply with the restraint regulations, one method of avoiding regulatory sanctions for noncompliance is for administrators and directors to examine the *Guidelines* and develop unique responses to the new requirements, taking into account the size and resources of the care facility.

For example, if 60% of a facility's residents are restrained, surveyors may conclude, on that basis alone, that the facility is deficient. Although under the *Guidelines* such a raw percentage itself should not lead to a deficiency, it would trigger a surveyor investigation of the documentation of each instance of restraint use.

Facilities must ensure that surveyors will find evidence that the facility is attempting to improve residents' quality of care and quality of life creatively and actively by the judicious and sparing use of physical and chemical restraints, used as a last resort rather than as standard practice, and even then only under well-documented circumstances. Examples of ways to limit exposure arising from restraint use are described in the next section.

Documentation of Restraint Use and Permission

The best way for a facility to avoid being cited for noncompliance with the OBRA '87 restraint requirement is to document painstakingly all instances of permission to use restraints and their subsequent use. The HCFA Guidelines state unequivocally that surveyors must be provided with documented evidence that caregivers attempted to use less restrictive solutions before using restraints, and that the decision to use restraints is the outcome of a medical decision involving a physical or occupational therapist. It is absolutely critical that facilities develop a "paper trail" for surveyors.

The nursing assessment and individualized care plans are the ideal vehicle through which nurses can perform a comprehensive assessment of the resident's potential for injury to self or others. The assessments identify reasons for behavioral and medical conditions, state whether the cause of the conditions can be treated, list alternate nursing interventions other than restraints, and estimate the amount of risk to the resident and others in the facility. One instrument a facility might use for this function is a checklist such as that shown in Figure 15.1.

Facilities should develop a grid that identifies at a glance the number and location of restrained residents. The type of restraint used should also be identified. Besides making restraint checks easier, such a grid may prompt staff members to consider whether a particular type of restraint is absolutely necessary for a particular resident or whether other interventions would substitute adequately for restraints.

Facilities also must begin a comprehensive review of medical orders for restrained residents to ensure that at all times a valid physician's order exists that specifies the circumstances and intervals during which restraints may be used. These orders should be transferred to a separate form to be maintained at the nurses' stations for ease of reference.

Finally, facilities should provide frequent in-service education for staff members concerning the correct way to tie restraints. A common mistake that nursing assistants make is to apply posey vests backwards. Facilities should take steps to ensure that this is one restraint accident that never occurs. Facilities should reinforce hands-on training with video training sessions that cover the procedures for the correct application of restraints and the circumstances under which restraints may be applied. Often, restraint manufacturers and distributors make training videos available to their customers.

Name: _____ Date: _____
Behavioral/medical condition: _____
Past history, including employment, habits, etc.: _____
_____
_____
_____

Past attempts to treat (place, dates of treatment, and duration of treatment): _____
_____
_____
_____
_____

Provided postural support? _____ Rearranged furniture? _____
Ensured staff continuity? _____ Individualized surroundings? _____
Lowered bed? _____

Risks (evaluate on a scale of 0 through 10):
To self: To others:
Falls _____   Abuse _____
Wandering _____
Self-mutilation _____

Figure 15.1.   Form for assessing a resident's potential for injury to self or others.

Less Restrictive Solutions to Particular Problems

Postural Support   The HCFA *Guidelines* require that a facility document its attempts to treat the resident using less restrictive methods before resorting to physical restraints. As mentioned, less restrictive measures include pillows, wedge cushions, pads, and lap trays that the resident is able to remove without assistance. Coupled with an exercise regimen, these measures may be effective in fostering proper body position, balance, and alignment and in helping to prevent contractures (HCFA, 1992, p. P-76). It is essential that facilities take seriously the necessity for precise documentation of attempts to use less restrictive measures, because the failure to do so will make facilities an easy target for surveyors.

Wandering   Caregivers should conduct a careful search for solutions to resident wandering. Placing rope or a yellow ribbon attached with Velcro across bedroom or exit doorways on a corridor may be enough to solve some problems. Installing sensitive alarm systems that can detect residents' attempts to leave the building may be necessary in larger facilities. It is important to note, however, that once a facility installs such a system, it must be diligent in ensuring that the system is operational and, as previous examples illustrate, that it is not disengaged for the convenience of staff.

One solution involves instructing staff members to assess residents' customary and usual lifetime habits. A resident may wander every day in response to the memory of a life-long routine. For example, a resident who wanders at night may have been a night watchman for many years and now may wander simply out of habit. Staff members might consider allowing the resident to walk at night, perhaps with the facility's security guard, until he is fatigued.

For residents who wander sporadically and are unable to recall the location of their bedroom, the dining area, or the restrooms, pasting colored shapes or colored objects on the doors to these areas may help residents remember which room is which, or at least provide an obvious guidepost. Another way to guide residents is to paint colored pathways or lay colored tiles in pathways that lead from bedrooms to central facility areas. The colors will catch residents' attention and may help them remember where they are going.

Facilities with residents who wander may find it helpful to have these residents wear identification bracelets that include the resident's name and the statement "Cognitively impaired—if lost, please call [the facility]." However, before the resident can be so identified, his or her family or legal representative must be consulted and must give the facility permission to identify the person in this or any other way that distinguishes him or her from other residents. Some facilities have attempted to identify residents who wander by attaching a piece of red cloth to the person's clothing—though, again, this may be done only with family permission—so that staff members can identify a potential problem easily and keep a close watch on the situation (Rader, 1987).

It is also possible to mark the medical charts of residents who wander for easy identification by staff members, and such a measure does not require special permission. However, all facility staff members should be made aware of the identity of residents who are likely to wander out of a facility. Not only the nurses, but also receptionists, housekeepers, and activity directors should be able to identify residents who may go outside and those who may not.

Adopting a policy for responding to residents who wander and educating every staff member as to the procedures to follow to locate residents are highly advisable steps that can be initiated easily.

These procedures should be reinforced with staff drills that focus on the fast, efficient location of wandering residents when necessary.

Staff Allocation Changes in staffing, not necessarily involving an increase, may smooth the transition to reduced restraint use. For example, most facilities currently schedule all personnel, except administrators, in three 8-hour shifts. It may be worthwhile to consider increasing staffing during the facility's busiest times. For example, if several residents wander at night, the facility might schedule more personnel at that time. During peak hours of the morning and late afternoon or evening, the facility might staff more heavily with part-time nurses' aides.

Some facilities make permanent staff-to-resident assignments, so that staff members and residents have more opportunity to build rapport and understanding. As a result, residents who sense continuity and routine may be less agitated and disoriented.

Facilities might also consider using nonnursing personnel more intensively. Having occupational therapists and physical therapists implement walking and exercise programs and allowing therapists to instruct nurses' aides on how to use these programs actually may reduce the number of nurses needed, because exercise can alleviate many conditions. An area outside the facility might even be enclosed where residents may walk, alone or accompanied by volunteers.

Falls Lowering beds is one way to reduce injuries resulting from falls. Although this practice could make the provision of nursing care too difficult if done facility-wide, it could be the ideal solution for the few residents who regularly fall out of bed. If lowering beds is not practicable, installing padding on the floor around the bed may prevent injuries if the resident does fall.

Furniture should be arranged so that a resident may use it for support as he or she moves from the bed to the bathroom. In some instances, such as for residents who otherwise would require assistance or a wheelchair in order to go to the bathroom, this measure may substantially decrease a resident's risk of experiencing a serious fall.

Drug Holidays and Drug Use Although in many instances drugs are used legitimately to treat older adults' physical ailments, drugs can have unpleasant side effects, even when properly prescribed and administered. Some facilities designate one day a month as a "drug holiday." On that day, no medication is administered except in emergency circumstances. This is an opportunity for residents' bodies to experience relief from constant medication.

The HCFA *Guidelines* contain in-depth instructions to surveyors for drug use review (DUR). Facilities should plan DUR programs that analyze potential problems, such as:

- Use of ineffective drugs
- Excessive dose
- Excessive duration of therapy
- Inadequate dose
- Inadequate duration of therapy
- Products more expensive than necessary
- Drug interactions
- Prescribing by multiple physicians
- Inadequate documentation (Sherman, 1989)

Establishing an effective DUR program requires that these steps be followed:

- Analyze facility needs and objectives for a DUR program
- Systematize data collection and analysis
- Develop drug use profiles
- Develop preestablished standards for drug prescribing and use
- Develop education programs for physicians, pharmacists, nurses, and residents
- Provide for program evaluation and program flexibility as changes in drug use occur (Sherman, 1989, p. 79)

A DUR program will enable a facility to identify residents who are taking medication for unspecified reasons. In addition, residents who require medication will be more likely to receive the proper drugs in the prescribed doses. Finally, an implemented DUR program that surveyors can observe in action may dramatically reduce a facility's exposure to deficiency citations that relate to residents' receiving medications as prescribed.

CREATING A RESTRAINT-FREE ENVIRONMENT

An increasing number of long-term care facilities throughout the United States are learning and adapting to restraint-free care, with some facilities even adopting a "restraint-free" policy. Facilities that have undertaken restraint-free care do report significant benefits, such as increased morale for both residents and staff. Research indicates that achieving a restraint-free environment is a goal that may not necessarily be attained; however, as providers aim to create a restraint-free environment, care alternatives can be developed for most residents for whom restraints are inappropriate.

Implementing a restraint-free policy requires reeducating and training the entire care facility staff: nursing, physical therapy, occupational therapy, in-service education, administration, maintenance, and housekeeping. Every staff member must be aware of and willing to implement the policy. It will probably be necessary to draw on all the available eyes and ears in the facility to keep track of the more active residents and those who wander.

The commitment to restraint-free care is one that will command all of the facility's resources. Nevertheless, the results that restraint-free facilities report are notable for their lack of injuries to residents. Facilities may use a restraint-free ideal to ensure that the reduced use of restraints mandated by OBRA '87 is actually achieved.

REVIEW OF FACILITY POLICIES AND PROCEDURES

Several courts that have imposed liability on facilities for restraint-related injuries have looked to the facility's own restraint and supervision policies and procedures to determine the standard of care (*Kujawski v. Arbor View Health Care Center*, 1987; *Stiffelman v. Abrams*, 1983). For example, federal regulations require that restraints be checked every 2 hours and that the resident be repositioned. However, some facilities have developed policies that require restraint checks every 30 minutes or every hour. Facilities should take great care to update facility policy and procedures to reflect the OBRA '87 changes. To the extent that their policy differs from the requirements set forth in OBRA '87, they should also employ special vigilance to ensure that the policy adopted by the facility represents a standard of care to which the facility is willing to be held.

CONCLUSION

Restraint reform measures present many challenges to long-term care providers. However, through a solid understanding of the substance and ramifications of these measures, providers can take affirmative steps to prepare for the increasingly stringent requirements for restraint use contained in OBRA '87 and state-level restraint reform measures. Adopting appropriate restraint policies and procedures and reeducating facility staff members to regard restraint use only as a last resort in care dilemmas can significantly reduce a facility's exposure to regulatory, civil, and criminal liability. Furthermore, by responding promptly to the social concerns about the appropriateness of restraint use that are embodied in these measures, providers may avoid the undue wrath of advocacy groups and the media as our nation comes to terms with the changing role of restraints.

REFERENCES

Avorn, J., Dryer, P., Connelly, K., & Soumerai, S. (1989). Use of psychoactive medication and the quality of care in rest homes. *New England Journal of Medicine, 260,* 227–232.

Beers, M., Avorn, J., Soumerai, S., Everitt, D., Sherman, D., & Salem, S. (1988). Psychoactive medication use in intermediate-care facility residents. *Journal of American Medical Association, 260,* 3016–3020, 3054.

Booty v. Kentwood Manor Nursing Home, Inc., 483 So.2d 634 (La. Ct. App. 1985)

Burns, B., & Kamerow, D. (1988). Psychotropic drug prescription for nursing home residents. *Journal of Family Practice, 26,* 155–160.

Cal. Code Regs. title 22, §72527(a) (8).

Cal. [Health & Safety] Code §1430(b) (Deering 1992).

Cal. [Welfare and Institutions] Code §15610(c) (6), 15632, 15634(d) (1900).

Cramer v. Theda Clark Memorial Hospital, 172 N.W.2d 427 (Wisc. 1970).

Dow v. State, 60 N.Y.S.2d 342, 183 Misc. 674 (1944).

Dusine v. Golden Shores Convalescent Center, Inc., 249 So.2d 40 (Fla. Dist. Ct. App. 1971).

Evans, L., & Strumpf, N. (1989). Tying down the elderly: A review of the literature on physical restraints. *Journal of American Geriatric Society, 37,* 65–74.

Farnsworth, E. (1973). Nursing homes use caution when they use restraints. *Modern Nursing Home, 30,* 4.

Fed. Reg. Code title 42, §483.10(b) (4), 483.10(d) (3), 483.13(a), 483.15(b), 483.15(m), 483.25, 483.25(c) (1), 483.25(e) (1), 483.25(e) (2), 483.25(h) (1), 483.25(1), 1991.

Federal Register, vol. 54, pp. 5321, 5323, 5360 (1989).

Fields v. Senior Citizens Center, Inc. of Coushatta, 428 So.2d 343 (La. Ct. App. 1988).

Fleming v. Prince George's County, 277 Md. 685, 358 A.2d 892 (1976).

Frengley, J., & Mion, L. (1986). Incidence of physical restraints on acute general medical wards. *Journal of American Geriatric Society, 34,* 565–568.

General Laws of Rhode Island, §23-17.8-1(b), 23-17.8-3(a), (b), (c), 23-17.8-10 (a)(1991).

Golden Villa Nursing, Inc. v. Smith, 674 S.W.2d 343 (Tex. Ct. App. 1984).

Green, W., & Pollack, J. (1990, March 26). Nursing home is liable in restraint case. *Wall Street Journal* (p. B5, col. 1).

Health Care Financing Administration. (1992). *Interpretative Guidelines, State Operations Manual,* Rev. 250.

Horton v. Niagara Falls Memorial Medical Center, 380 N.Y.S.2d 116, 51 A.D.2d 152 (N.Y. App. Div. 1976).

Juhnke v. Evangelical Lutheran Good Samaritan Soc'y., 634 P.2d 1132 (Kan. Ct. App. 1981).

Kujawski v. Arbor View Health Care Center, 139 Wis. 2d 455, 407 N.W.2d 249 (1987).

McGillivray v. Rapides Iberia Management Enterprises, 493 So.2d 819 (La. Ct. App. 1986).

Md. Code Ann., [Health—General] §19-1405 (1992).

Missouri Annotated Statutes, §199.088, 1983.

Morningside Hospital & Training School for Nurses v. Pennington, 189 Okla. 170, 114 P.2d 943 (1941).

New York Consolidated Law Service, Public Health, §12(1), 12-b, 12-b(2), 1989.

New York Times. (1989, Dec. 28). p. 1, col. 1.

Nichols v. Green Acres Rest Home, Inc., 245 So.2d 544 (La. Ct. App. 1971).

Northrup v. Archbishop Bergan Mercy Hospital, 575 F.2d 605 (8th Cir. 1978).

Nursing Home Community Coalition of New York State (1989).

Omnibus Budget Reconciliation Act of 1987. Pub. L. No. 100-203, 101 Stat. 1330.

People v. Coe, 71 N.Y.2d 852, 522 N.E.2d 1039, 527 N.Y.S.2d 741 (1988).

Rader, J. (1987). A comprehensive staff approach to wandering. *Gerontologist, 27,* 756–760.

Restatement (Second) of Torts, §319 (1965).

Rubenstein, H., Miller, F., Postel, S., & Evans, H. (1983). Standards of medical care based on consensus rather than evidence: The case of routine bedrail use for the elderly. *Law, Medicine and Health Care, 11,* 271.

Rudder, C. (1989, July). *Psychotropic drug use with New York State nursing home residents, 4,* Nursing Home Community Coalition of New York State.

Sherman, S. (1989, August). Drug utilization review in long term care. *Contemporary Long Term Care,* 79–80.

Stiffelman v. Abrams, 655 S.W.2d 528 (Mo. 1983).

U.S.C.A. title 42, §1320a-7a, 1396r(h) (1) (B), 1396r(h) (2) (B) (i), 1396r(h) (3) (C) (i), 1396r(h) (3) (C) (ii) 12 (1992).

Chapter 16

Ethical Issues Affecting the Use of Restraints

Steven Lipson

The inappropriate and sometimes abusive use of physical and chemical restraints has received much attention. Although on rare occasions restraints may have been used with the intent of inflicting harm, for the most part restraints have been used in long-term care facilities because staff believed that they helped protect frail residents from hurting themselves or that they were the only means of providing appropriate care. Thus, residents who fell frequently were tied down so that they could not hurt themselves. Residents who were agitated and at risk of harming themselves or others were given tranquilizers, or tied to a chair. A consensus developed that using restraints reflected the appropriate standard of care for residents in long-term care settings.

Although restraints are still considered effective and widely used in hospitals, their use in long-term care facilities has been questioned and heavily regulated. The evidence now suggests that restraints do not prevent injuries and can, moreover, cause injury. Some advocates have argued that informed consent should be required before physical restraints are used, since they may be considered "investigational or nonvalidated therapy" (Moss & La Puma, 1991).

THE CONFLICT BETWEEN
BENEFICENCE AND RESPECT FOR AUTONOMY

Workers at all levels of health care are assumed to operate in accordance with the principle of *beneficence*, which suggests that caregivers always act in the best interests of the patient or resident. Caregivers are expected to try to preserve life and to reduce pain and suffering to the best of their ability.

Until very recently, caregivers were expected to act paternalistically—that is, they were supposed to know what was best for the patient and resident and to take whatever action was needed. In the nursing home, this meant that treatments and medications were ordered without the knowledge or consent of the residents. In many states, nursing home administrators were even allowed to sign consent for residents to have surgery.

Since the 1970s, a new view of the respective roles of the resident and caregiver has evolved that gives the resident a greater role in his or her care. The 1987 OBRA regulations, the Residents' Bill of Rights and the Patient Self-Determination Act (see Appendixes 16.A and 16.B) reflect this new respect for the autonomy of the resident. Today, nursing home residents must be informed of their condition, must be allowed to participate in planning their care, and must be allowed to refuse treatment. The paternalistic attitude that once prevailed has been replaced. Caregivers may no longer restrict the freedom of their patients by ordering courses of treatment that the patient or resident chooses not to undergo. According to Collopy (1992),

> Respect for autonomy means respect for the right of individuals to shape *their own* lives in terms of their own values and goals, in accord with their own insights and limitations, and despite the risks and unpredictabilities that can accompany any course of human choice and action.

Respecting the autonomy of the nursing home resident does not relieve caregivers of the obligation to act beneficently, and difficult moral choices often arise when different rights and values become pitted against one another in the clinical setting. The case studies that follow illustrate how caregivers must consider the rights of the resident in making decisions that affect their care:

> Mr. Smith, an 83-year-old man with advanced Parkinson's disease, was admitted to the nursing home following the death of his caregiver. Despite regular monitoring of his medication by his physician, Mr. Smith fell frequently while at home. Mr. Smith's daughter is very worried that her father will break his hip and become bedbound, and asks the staff to restrict her father's movements so that he will not fall again. In order both to protect Mr. Smith from injuring himself and to respect his autonomy, the staff must look for a way to prevent Mr. Smith from falling without interfering with his activities. They must try to find an approach that is acceptable to him.

Mrs. Jones, a 79-year-old woman, was admitted to the nursing home from a local hospital following a severe stroke. She is paralyzed on her left side and is unable to write, speak, or make signs to communicate. During her hospital stay, she was given large doses of a sedating tranquilizer (Ativan) which made her very lethargic, because her constant calling out disrupted the unit. Now that she is in the nursing home, the staff must find a way of dealing with her calling out which does not reduce her level of consciousness.

Mrs. Lewis has lived in the facility for 3 years. Recently, she has refused to take her antihypertensive medication on the grounds that it is too expensive and constipates her. The nursing staff worry that without this drug, Mrs. Lewis is likely to have a stroke and possibly die. They have been unable to convince her to take her medicine. They meet with the physician and the pharmacist to determine whether a less expensive medication that will not slow her bowel function can be substituted.

All of these cases reveal the conflict between the obligation to the resident based on beneficence, on the one hand, and the need to respect the resident's autonomy, on the other. This conflict demands that alternatives to physical and chemical restraints, as described elsewhere in this book, be sought.

RESOLVING ETHICAL CONFLICTS

Finding solutions to care problems such as those described by the cases of Mr. Smith, Mrs. Jones, and Mrs. Lewis may be made more difficult by conflicting values. Each of us has values and beliefs by which we give meaning to the world and our experience of it, including: 1) the experience of illness, disease, injury, pain, and suffering and 2) the reality and eventual imminence of our death (McCullough & Lipson, 1989). Mr. Smith's daughter may feel that it is more important to make sure that her father does not break his hip than it is to preserve his dignity. Mrs. Jones' family may insist that Ativan be discontinued, since it appears to add to her confusion. Yet without the medication she yells constantly and disturbs her roommate. How can we resolve these conflicts without acting paternalistically, that is, without forcing the different parties to accept our decisions?

The first step in resolving ethical conflicts such as these is to examine the sources from which they arise. Sometimes conflicts are based on a misunderstanding or lack of knowledge. In other cases, conflict arises from a difference in values. Some residents have a very strong need to remain independent, and are willing to accept serious risks in order to do so. Other residents want to avoid pain and suffering at almost any cost. Yet other residents want to stay alive, regardless of the level of disability or pain that may be involved. In order to respect the individual's autonomy, it is important to know how the resident and his or her family rank these different goals. Sometimes, caregivers find that there is agreement over values, making compromise over decisions easier.

Physicians, administrators, ethicists, and members of the care team should ask the following questions to try to resolve ethical conflicts:

1. What are the facts of the situation? Do all parties have the same information? In the case of Mr. Smith, is the daughter aware of the research showing that restraints are not effective in preventing falls, and are often associated with increased injuries?

2. What are the responsibilities to the resident under the principles of beneficence and respect for autonomy? In the case of Mrs. Jones, administering a drug that increases the resident's confusion is not in that resident's best interest. Since the resident herself is unable to communicate her desires, Mrs. Jones' family should be consulted as to whether Mrs. Jones ever expressed her wishes on treatment rather than asking what they want done.

3. What are our responsibilities to other parties, such as families, other residents, and regulatory authorities? In the case of Mrs. Jones, caregivers clearly have a responsibility to Mrs. Jones' roommate to provide an environment that does not cause her distress, or adversely affect her health.

4. Is there a convergence of responsibilities? Does the principle of respect for autonomy or that of beneficence make one approach to resolving the conflict better than another? Since no rule states that one principle takes precedence over another, careful evaluation of each situation is crucial. In the case of Mr. Smith, if the staff can find a way to reduce the risk of falling while maintaining his feelings of independence by walking him to meals and activities, they will have addressed their obligations under both principles.

5. If no resolution of a conflict can be found, what values underlie the failure to resolve the conflict? It is sometimes effective to have the participants in an ethical conflict step back from what they think are the "right" answers and consider what it is they are trying to accomplish. It may be that once Mr. Smith's daughter realizes that preserving her father's functioning is best accomplished by maintaining his muscle strength and coordina-

tion by allowing him to walk, her enthusiasm over having her father restrained will wane.

CONCLUSION

As long-term care facilities move toward more resident-centered care and focus more on the respect for autonomy and the need to preserve the dignity of residents, the use of restraints has become increasingly unacceptable. The use of restraints is inconsistent with a philosophy of care that stresses the self-determination of residents and communication between residents and caregivers, and is thus inappropriate ethically. Caregivers must seek alternatives to restraint use, so that the resident's right to autonomy and dignity is preserved.

REFERENCES

Collopy, B.J. (1992). *The use of restraints in long-term care: The ethical issues.* White Paper. Washington, DC: American Association of Homes for the Aging.

Collopy, B., Boyle, P., & Jennings, B. (1991). New directions in nursing home ethics. *Hastings Center Report, 2,* 1–15.

Concern for Dying. (undated). *Advance directive protocols and the patient self-determination act.* New York, 1.

McCullough, L.B., & Lipson, S. (1989). A framework for geriatric ethics. In W. Reichel, Ed., *Clinical aspects of aging,* 3rd ed. (pp. 577–586). Baltimore: Williams & Wilkins.

Montgomery County Government Department of Family Resources. (undated). *Do you have questions or concerns about nursing homes?* Wheaton, MD: Montgomery County Government.

Moss, R.J., & La Puma, J. (1991). The ethics of mechanical restraints. *Hastings Center Report, 21*(1), 22–25.

Appendix 16.A

Residents' Bill of Rights

Residents of nursing facilities have special rights under federal and state law:

- Dignity, respect and courtesy
- Freedom from mental and physical abuse
- Freedom from chemical or physical restraint unless authorized by a physician
- A total care plan and complete information about facility services and charges
- Access to a personal physician and to medical information about diagnosis and treatment, with freedom to accept or refuse such treatment
- Presentation of grievances and suggestions without fear of reprisal
- A reasonable response to requests from facility administrator and staff
- Privacy: in resident's medical care program and room; in visits and communications; and in receipt of mail
- Management of personal finances unless otherwise designated by resident
- Secure storage and use of personal clothing and possessions
- Refusal to perform services for facility without resident's consent and approval of personal physician
- Thirty days advance written notice of discharge describing reasons for decision and appeal rights. A resident may not be transferred or discharged except for medical reasons, his own or other residents' welfare or for non-payment. A medicaid-certified facility must consider medicaid reimbursement as payment in full.

Source: Montgomery County Government Department of Family Resources.

Appendix 16.B

The Patient Self-Determination Act

The Patient Self-Determination Act (PSDA) took effect on December 1, 1991. It applies to hospitals, skilled nursing facilities, home health agencies, hospice organizations and health maintenance organizations which serve Medicare and Medicaid patients.

The PSDA requires these institutions to develop and maintain written policies and procedures to provide written information to adults to whom the institutions provide care. This written material must describe:

- an individual's rights under state law (including both statutory and case law) to make decisions about medical care, including the right to accept or refuse medical and surgical treatment;
- an individual's rights under state law to formulate advance medical directives such as a living will or durable power of attorney for health care, to guide the provision of care when the individual is incapacitated;
- the policies and procedures that the institution has developed to honor these rights.

Adapted from *Advance directive protocols and the patient self-determination act.* New York: Concern for Dying.

Suggested Readings

Activity Programming

Beisgen, B. (1989). *Life enhancing activities for mentally impaired elders*. New York: Springer Publishing.

Bloom, J. (1980). Withdrawal in the agency and what can be done about it. *Geriatric Care Newsletter, 12*(5).

Coons, D. (1991). *Specialized dementia care units*. Baltimore: Johns Hopkins University Press.

Cusack, O., & Smith, E. (1984). *Pets and the elderly, the therapeutic bond*. Special issue of *Activities, Adaptation and Aging, 4*(2/3). New York: Haworth Press.

Foster, P. (Ed.). (1986). *Therapeutic activities with the impaired elderly*. Special issue of *Activities, Adaptation and Aging, 8*(3/4). New York: Haworth Press.

Greenblatt, F. (1988). *Therapeutic recreation for long-term care facilities*. New York: Human Services Press.

Gwyther, L. (1985). *Care of Alzheimer's patients: A manual for nursing home staff*. Washington, DC: Alzheimer's Disease and Related Disorders Association.

Hastings, L. (1981). *Complete handbook of activities and recreational programs for nursing homes*. Englewood Cliffs, NJ: Prentice Hall.

Karras, B. (Ed.). (1987). *You bring out the music in me: Music in Nursing homes*. Special issue of *Activities, Adaptation and Aging, 10*(1/2). New York: Haworth Press.

Lake, J., & Williams, J. (1984). *Educational activity programs for older adults: A 12-month idea guide for adult education instructors and activity directors in gerontology*. New York: Haworth Press.

Martin-Erkison, L., & Leide, C. (1981). *Remembering automobiles, remembering trains*. Blue Mounds, WI: Bi-Folkal Productions.

Nolan, N. (1987). Activity programming for withdrawn confused residents. *Activities, Adaptation and Aging, 9*(4). New York: Haworth Press.

Peckham, C., & Peckham, A. (1982). *Activities keep me going*. Nashville: Parthenon Press.

Zgola, J. (1987). *Doing things: A guide to programming activities for persons with Alzheimer's disease and related disorders*. Baltimore: Johns Hopkins University Press.

Ethics of Restraint Use

Collopy, B., Boyle, P. & Jennings, B. (1990). New directions in nursing home ethics. *Hastings Center Report, 21*(2), 1–15.

Kapp, M.B. (1991). Reducing restraint use in nursing homes: The governing board's role. *Quality Review Bulletin, 17*(1), 22–25.

Levenson, S.A. (1989). Ethical and humanistic considerations in the care of the elderly. In W. Reichel (Ed.), Clinical aspects of aging (3rd ed.) (pp. 522–532). Baltimore: Williams & Wilkins.

Strumpf, N.E., & Evans, L.K. (1991). The ethical problems of prolonged physical restraint. *Journal of Gerontological Nursing, 17*(2), 22–30.

Use of Physical Restraints

Bauer, A., & Roedel, R. (1991, April). Successful restraint reduction techniques. *Contemporary Long Term Care, 48*, 50, 74.

Cutchins, C. (1991, July). Blueprint for restraint-free care. *American Journal of Nursing*, 36–44.

Evans, L.K., & Strumpf, N.E. (1989). Tying down the elderly. *Journal of the American Geriatrics Society, 37*, 65-74.

Evans, L.K., & Strumpf, N.E. (1990). Myths about elder restraint. *Image, 22*(2), 124–127.

Feutz-Harter, S.A. (1990). Legal implications of restraints. *Journal of Nursing Administration, 20*(10), 8–9.

Gold, M.F. (1991). Moving away from restraints, *Provider*, 20–29.

Harper, C., & Lyles, Y. (1988). Physiology and complications of bedrest. *Journal of the American Geriatrics Society, 36*(11), 1047–1054.

Hegland, A. (1991, April). Restraint removal: Old habits die hard. *Contemporary Long Term Care, 35*–36, 70–71, 87.

Johnson, S.H. (1990). The fear of liability and the use of restraints in nursing homes. *Law, Medicine and Health Care, 18*(3), 263–273.

Jones, L.F. (1990, March). Progressive restraint release without additional staffing. *Contemporary Long Term Care*, 60–61.

Lofgren, R., MacPherson, D., Granieri, R., Myllenbeck, S., & Sttafka, J. (1989). Mechanical restraints on the medical wards: Are protective devices safe? *American Journal of Public Health, 79*(6), 735–738.

Masters, R., & Marks, S. (1990). The use of restraints. *Rehabilitation Nursing, 15*(1), 22–25.

Mion, L.C., Frengley, J.D., Jakovic, C.A., & Marino, J.A. (1989). A further exploration of the use of physical restraints in hospitalized patients. *Journal of the American Geriatrics Society, 37*, 949–956.

Moss, R.J., & LaPuma, J. (1991). The ethics of mechanical restraints. *Hastings Center Report, 21*(1), 22–25.

Neary, M.A., Kanski, G., Janelli, L., Scherer, Y., & North, N. (1991, July/August). Restraints as nurse's aides see them. *Geriatric Nursing*, 191–192.

Powell, C., Mitchell-Pedersen, L., Fingerote, E., & Edmund, L. (1989). Freedom from restrants: Consequences of reducing physical restraints in the management of the elderly. *Canadian Medical Association Journal, 27*(6), 756–760.

Rader, J. (1987). A comprehensive staff approach to problem wandering. *Gerontologist, 27*(6), 756–760.

Rajecki, R. (1990, January). Reducing restraint reliance. *Contemporary Long Term Care*, 52–57.

Robbins, L. Boyko, E., Lane, J., Cooper, D., & Jahnigan, D. (1987). Binding the elderly: A prospective study in an acute care hospital. *Journal of the American Geriatrics Society, 35*(4), 290–296.

Schaefer, A., & Phil, D. (1985). Restraints in the elderly: When safety and autonomy conflict. *Canadian Medical Association Journal, 132,* 1257–1260.

Strumpf, N.E., & Evans, L.K. (1988). Physical restraint of the hospitalized eldery: Perceptions of patients and nurses. *Nursing Research, 37*(3), 132–137.

Strumpf, N.E., Evans, L.K., & Schwartz, D. (1990, May/June). Restraint-free care: From dream to reality. *Geriatraic Nursing, 11*(3), 122–124.

Suprock, L.A. (1990, November/December). Changing the rules. *Geriatric Nursing, 11*(6), 288–289.

Tinetti, M. (1987). Factors associated with serious injury during falls by ambulatory nursing home residents. *Journal of the American Geriatrics Society, 35*(7), 644–648.

Werner, P., Cohen-Mansfield, J., Braun, J., & Marx, M. (1989). Physical restraints and agitation in nursing home residents. *Journal of the American Geriatrics Society, 37,* 1122–1126.

Williams, C.C. (1989). The experience of long term care in the future. *Journal of Gerontological Social Work, 14,* 3–18.

Use of Psychoactive Drugs

Avorn, J., Dreyer, P., Connelly, K., & Soumerai, S.B. (1989). Use of psychoactive medication and the quality of care in rest homes. *New England Journal of Medicine, 320*(4), 227–232.

Beers, M. Avorn, J., Soumerai, S.B., Everett, D.E., Sherman, D.S., & Salem, S. (1988). *Journal of the American Medical Association, 260*(20), 3016–3020.

Cooper, J.W., (1989). Use of chemical restraints in nursing homes. *Nursing Homes,* 5–7.

Feinberg, J.L. (1990). Nonpharmacologic alternatives to chemical restraints. *Consultant Pharmacist, 5*(7), 380–386.

Gerrard, J. et al. (1991). Evaluation of neuroleptic drug use by nursing home elderly under proposed Medicare and Medicaid regulations. *Journal of the American Medical Association, 265*(4), 463–476.

Grossberg, G.T. et al. (1990). Psychiatric problems in the nursing home. *Journal of the American Geriatrics Society, 38*(5), 542–552.

Gurwitz, J.H., Soumerai, S.B., & Avorn, J. (1990). Improving medication prescribing and utilization in the nursing home. *Journal of the American Geriatrics Society, 38*(5), 542–552.

Johnson, J. (1990). Evaluating psychotropic drug use in the nursing home. *Provider,* 36–37.

Stephenson, D. (1990). Medication restraints. *Geriatric Health Care Review, 1*(6), 1–4.

Index